The Firefly Project

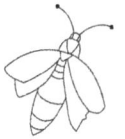

Conversations about what it means to be alive

Perspectives in Medical Humanities

Perspectives in Medical Humanities publishes scholarship produced or reviewed under the auspices of the University of California Medical Humanities Consortium, a multi-campus collaborative of faculty, students and trainees in the humanities, medicine, and health sciences. Our series invites scholars from the humanities and health care professions to share narratives and analysis on health, healing, and the contexts of our beliefs and practices that impact biomedical inquiry.

General Editor

Brian Dolan, PhD, Professor of Social Medicine and Medical Humanities
University of California, San Francisco (UCSF)

First published in 2013
by the University of California Medical Humanities Press
San Francisco

© 2013
University of California
Medical Humanities Consortium
3333 California Street, Suite 485
San Francisco, CA 94143-0850

Cover Art by Sherri Corron

Library of Congress Control Number: 2013934055

isbn 978-0-9889865-0-3

Printed in USA

www.medicalhumanities.ucsf.edu | brian.dolan@ucsf.edu

This book series is made possible by the generous support of the Dean of the School of Medicine at UCSF, the Center for Humanities and Health Sciences at UCSF, and a Multicampus Center Research Program grant from the University of California Office of the President.

To my husband Fred Lurmann, and our children
Amy, David, Kaitlin, with great love;

To Ernest H. Rosenbaum, MD,
who believed in me from the very beginning;

For all the patients through the years
who have inspired us with their stories;

For all of the young people whose loving attention
helped those stories emerge;

and

In loving memory of all the patients
whose lives graced our program until they died.

It is believed that the souls
of ordinary people take the
shapes of spiders,
while those of heroes appear in
the form of fireflies.

This publication would not have been possible without the generous support of Mount Zion
Health Fund of the Jewish Community Endowment Fund.

Cynthia D. Perlis, Director
Art for Recovery
UCSF Helen Diller Family Comprehensive Cancer Center
1600 Divisadero Street
San Francisco, CA 94115
415.885.7221
Cynthia.Perlis@ucsfmedctr.org
http://cc.ucsf.edu/afr

Table of Contents

One: An Unplanned Life

Two: Knock On Wood

Three: The Space Between

Four: Whisper In My Soul

Five: Epilogue

Foreword

We are delighted to include The Firefly Project in the Perspectives in Medical Humanities publication series. As we go into our second year of publications, the scholarship and creative works produced by the University of California Medical Humanities Press have helped to define the emergent field of medical humanities. Our authors – medical practitioners, patients, poets, scientists, scholars and artists – collectively demonstrate how different voices and visions of healthcare broaden our understanding of health and illness. Celebrating its twentieth anniversary, the Firefly Project fosters dialogue and explores different perceptions of illness through the writings of cancer patients and students. The present book not only complements our endeavors to find new meaning in how we cope with disease, but adds a unique perspective through its form of literary expression: excerpts from correspondence between patients and pen pals.

The authors represented here were participants in the Firefly Project, a component of Art for Recovery, an innovative and unique program at the UCSF Helen Diller Family Comprehensive Cancer Center. The project connects patients, medical students and community teenagers through a monthly exchange of written correspondence and a collaborative creative project. Not emails, not tweets, not blog postings, but good old-fashioned letters sent through the mail. The letter writers become practitioners in what we have called "slow communication," preserving the art of forming relationships through crafting meaningful exchanges over time. The aim of the project is to give patients coping with life-threatening illness the opportunity to express their feelings through thoughtful writing and to become teachers and mentors by sharing their experience. Students engage in a reflective dialogue to help them better understand patients' concerns, needs and preferences in discussing their lives and illness and what the world of medicine is beginning to mean to them. The letters also to give them an opportunity to write about their own personal losses.

Over 3,000 people have participated in the Firefly Project since its inception, the history of which is further discussed in the introduction to this volume. The director of Art for Recovery, Cynthia Perlis, selected the excerpts from this archive of letters. Individually, they provide touching and engaging insights into how people learn to talk about disease and the impact of illness on their lives. Collectively, they tell us not only about disease

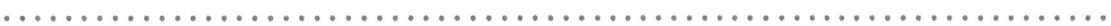

itself, or attitudes about the healthcare delivery system, or visceral reactions to treatment, but also about the journey of rediscovery of oneself and the transformation of identity created by the illness experience. It is an honor to share these insights with our readers.

~ Brian Dolan, PhD
Director of the University of California Medical Humanities Consortium
General Editor, Perspectives in Medical Humanities

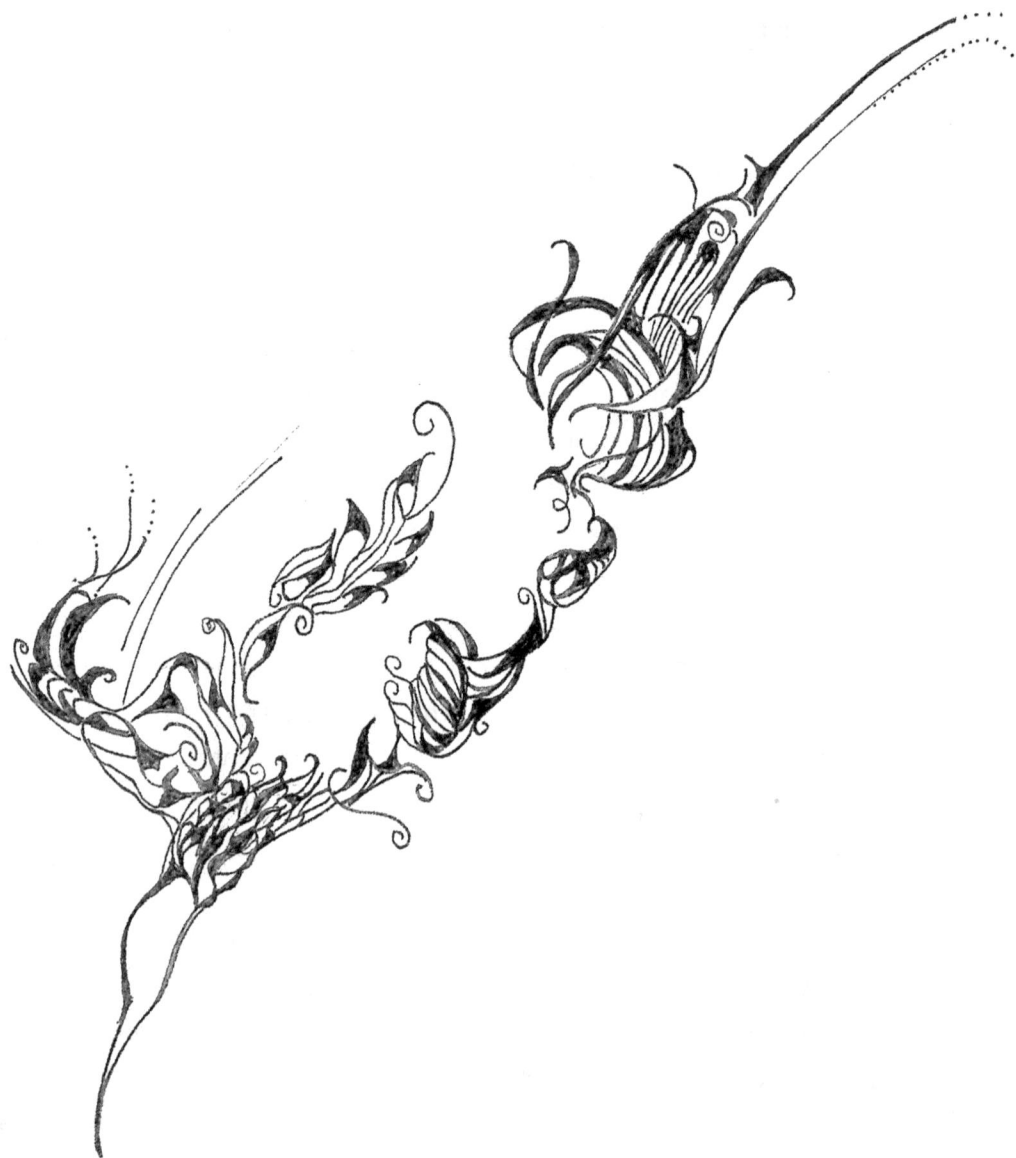

Introduction

In the beginning, in 1988, I was told to wear a mask, gloves and a gown when I entered a patient's room. I must disinfect the art supplies after each use. There was no cure for AIDS, and most died a terrible death while facing wasting disease, or Kaposi Sarcoma, loneliness and isolation. Nurses and doctors were getting needle sticks and running frantically down the hall, afraid their own health might become compromised. Fear was contagious. The hospital felt like a war zone. As I entered the rooms of these very young patients, mostly men, who were dying of AIDS, I asked them to tell me their story. I asked them if they were afraid of dying. At first they looked at me strangely. I was giving them permission to talk about fear or anger or death, something no one had granted them. Everyone else advised them to keep a positive attitude, and everything would be all right. Their minds and bodies could not accept this advice. There was no cure. There was very little hope. When I witnessed their distress, I took off my mask and gloves, and I held their hands. These young men wanted to be heard, to be touched and to be understood. They wanted to be treated like all human beings deserved to be treated. While I sat at their bedside, they began to create images on paper that told their own very personal story. Some of the drawings were very primitive; others were amazingly complex. All of them were powerful expressions about what it felt like to be dying of AIDS. I knew this is where I was meant to be. I was not afraid.

My father died suddenly of a cerebral hemorrhage when I was two years old. He was 35. I have no idea what his voice sounded like or what it might have felt like to have him hold me. I have no physical sense of him whatsoever except from photographs. My mother told me stories about what he was like, his interests and hobbies. From photographs, I knew that I had his thick brown hair and his dark brown eyes. My mother told me he was the kindest man she had ever met, the love of her life. She also told me that he was watching over me and protecting me. When I walked to school and looked up at the sky, I felt he was always there with me.

My mother went to work every day to support her three children. She did what she needed to do to provide a roof over our heads. She never learned to drive.

She took the bus everywhere while starting her own business and became a very successful business woman. Independent and hardworking, my mother did not expect anyone to help her. We were a different kind of family; no one I knew lived without a father. However, it was not until I was much older that I realized we were different. As the youngest, I was a latchkey kid. To me it was perfectly normal to come home every afternoon and wait alone until my sister and brother arrived. I drew and colored on anything that was available: paper, newspaper, napkins. My mother came home exhausted from long days at work, but every evening she sat down and asked me to tell her a story about my drawings. I loved that time with her. I felt heard and seen.

When folks ask me about Art for Recovery and how the Firefly Project was conceived, I realize now that I wanted to give to my patients (and the students who participate in Firefly) an opportunity to express their hopes and dreams, anger and fear. I wanted to give them what my mother had given me: recognition and a sense of value as a creative soul. She listened to me without judgment and always made me feel that I could express myself fully and completely. I wanted to give my patients a place where art-making, writing, music and poetry were available to them in a safe community of people going through similar experiences. I wanted to give them what the young men dying of AIDS in 1988 didn't have – a voice.

I remember those years in the HIV unit when young men preparing to die came to the hospital with quilts and rocking chairs. I remember their spirits when I walk the hallways today. When I look at the art they created, I remember their humor, their fear, their anger. I remember their dying. I remember each unique person by name and personality. This work has given me deep wounds and scars that heal slowly over time. It has given me painful memories. It has also given me great life affirming joy and the knowledge that we all have the potential to make a difference simply by being present. It has given me hope that people who feel isolated and alone or live in the darkest moments of illness and adversity, or are students looking for a way to give back because of their advantage and privilege, are inspired to connect with another human being, revealing their heart and soul.

I am incredibly grateful to Dr. Ernest H. Rosenbaum for hiring me in 15 minutes in 1988. I am grateful that I took a leap of faith and found myself on the HIV unit where no one survived in those days, but where I learned what it means to be alive and what it means to die. Those lessons will stay with me forever. I am grateful that Art for Recovery is the vessel that holds beautiful art work and written conversations about what it means to be healthy and sick, afraid and courageous, forgotten and remembered, poised at the brink of life, facing down death.

I thank my mother, the first person to believe in me, who taught me I had a responsibility as an artist to give my art to the world and to involve others in that process. I thank Dr. Ernest Rosenbaum for believing that Mount Zion Hospital was the place to do that. My mother gave me the gift of life, and Dr. Rosenbaum gave me the opportunity of a lifetime.

~ Cynthia D. Perlis
Director, Art for Recovery
Founder of The Firefly Project

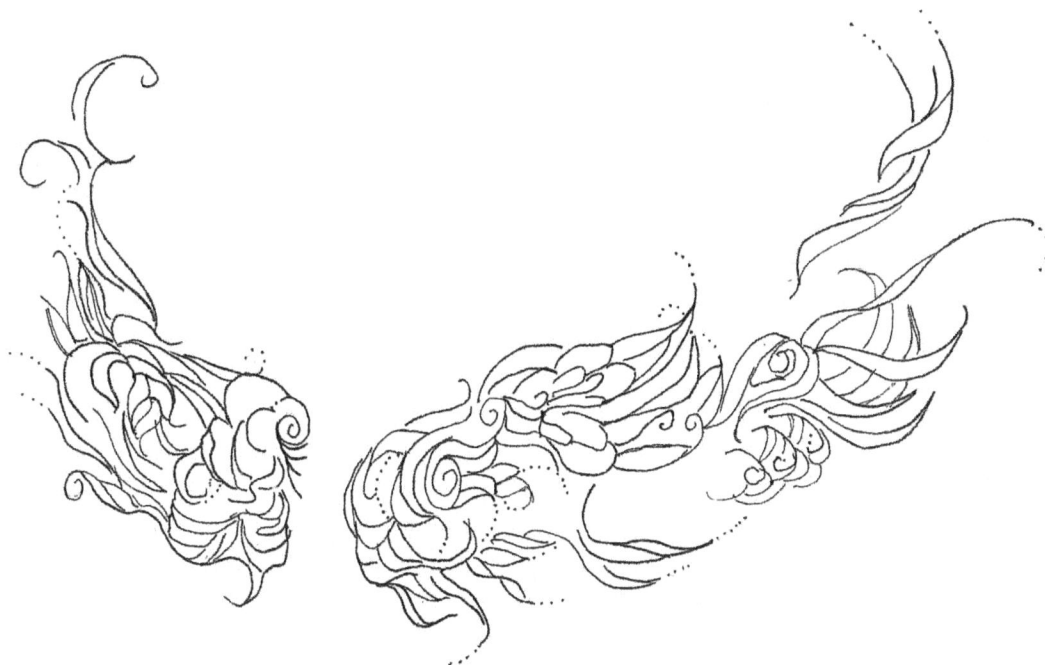

About Art for Recovery & The Firefly Project

The Firefly Project is one component of the Ernest H. Rosenbaum, MD, Art for Recovery program, an award-winning department of the UCSF Helen Diller Family Comprehensive Cancer Center. Art for Recovery brings artists, writers, musicians and medical students to the patients of the UCSF Medical Center to encourage them to express their pain, anger, hopes and dreams through images and words and music. Consistent with the mission of the University of California, San Francisco Medical Center – Caring, Healing, Teaching, Discovering, our aim is to give patients coping with life-threatening illness the opportunity to express their deepest feelings through creative experiences.

In 1988, Dr. Rosenbaum founded Art for Recovery out of a deep conviction that patients could better heal, cope with their illness and enjoy a better quality of life by engaging in the expressive arts. I have directed the program since its inception.

The Firefly Project evolved from my experiences as a privileged listener at the bedsides of those coping with cancer, AIDS and other diseases. As I listened to their life experiences and achievements unfold, it occurred to me that their stories needed to be shared, and these patients – so often hidden away, put on disability, avoided, isolated or otherwise marginalized during their illness – could become mentors and teachers of empathy and compassion. Patients share this vulnerable time in their lives, trying to understand their new identity as they go through physical and emotional changes and try to understand the new normal. Listeners grow in compassion and understanding as they look for common ground with those who are ill.

While working with the patients, I often told my own young teenagers about the lives of the patients I met at the bedside each day. These people were often identified by their disease rather than as people with vibrant histories. My kids did not care about why these people were in the hospital; they wanted to know about their life experiences. If my own kids were interested, I thought there must be hundreds of teenagers who wondered what it is like to be hospitalized and what these peoples' lives were like before they became *patients*. I thought about how much teenagers and adult patients have in common: feelings of dependence, isolation, being misunderstood, angst and loneliness. In addition, many teens have experienced personal loss.

How amazing it would be if they could express their feelings through writing to someone they have never met. How fantastic it would be for them to pour their hearts out to a stranger. Most importantly, teens could learn about compassion and empathy and focus on someone else rather than exclusively on their own thoughts and concerns. I also knew that the patients were eager to give something back, to share their life experiences and the wisdom that illness had taught them. Rather than being labeled "sick", they wanted to feel productive. It made perfect sense to bring these groups together, to shed light on two somewhat misunderstood, invisible populations. I wanted the richness and depth of their lives to become more public and accessible.

In 1992, The Firefly Project was born. The program pairs healthy teenagers, UCSF medical, nursing and pharmacy students with adults coping with life-threatening illness in a monthly exchange of letters and artwork throughout the school year. Participating students are given the opportunity to choose their pen pal through a brief description at the beginning of the year, and they write the first letter. Often there is hesitation about what to say or not say, especially in the first letter exchange. Eventually everyone finds his or her own comfort level and responds accordingly. In some instances, cancer is never mentioned; in most letters, however, people write about personal experiences of loss, cancer, teenage life or dealing with the complexities of medical school. Sometimes there is a suggestion from a student to a patient: "If you wish not to write about your cancer, you don't have to."

Because art-making is an important component of Art for Recovery, we ask the pen pals to collaborate on an art project during the school year. This can be whatever patient and student agree upon. Some create collages that are begun by a student, then added onto by a patient and completed by year's end. Some write short stories paragraph by paragraph, sent back and forth, until at year's end an entire essay is complete. Some create an altered book, where each participant alters the same book for the length of the project.

All correspondence goes through the office of Art for Recovery. No personal information (last names, addresses, etc.) is given out. At the end of the school year, pen pals meet for the first time during an Art for Recovery-facilitated healing service.

The excitement when folks meet for the first time after exchanging letters, sight unseen for an entire school year, lights up the room. In those first few moments of finally being together, there is a realization that the image writers held of their pen pal may not necessarily match the way they look in real life.

As the letters come in to the Art for Recovery office, I begin reading through them, selecting conversations which are provocative, questioning and filled with curiosity. These conversations are adapted into a script which is shared in a public reading or Adaptation a few weeks after the healing service. The actual pen pals then read "script in hand" to a community audience. I stand in awe of what these amazing people create together in the course of one school year.

A few years after the Firefly Project began, a palliative care physician came to the end-of-year Adaptation. She mentioned to me that her first- and second-year medical students were having a difficult time interviewing patients. She thought it would be interesting for them to "interview" the patients through letter writing, asking any questions they wished about details of the illness and how someone actually lived with a life-threatening diagnosis. When I approached the patients at the beginning of the year with the possibility of exchanging letters with a medical, pharmacy or nursing student, they loved the idea. Suddenly they became teachers of illness, describing what their experience had been as they worked with physicians to find treatments that worked or were disappointed as treatments were not successful. Currently, there are so many medical students who wish to participate in the Firefly Project that we have to turn many away.

Why does this project remain so popular year after year? Patients move beyond images of themselves as ill or disabled and discover they have much to give back. They find new purpose and meaning in their lives as they become teachers and mentors for their teenage pen pals. They are reconnected with their past in healing ways, remembering what it was like to be a teenager, rediscovering old interests, reviving forgotten self-images.

Thousands of students and patients have participated in the Firefly Project. Many of the patients have died – a few during the school year while participating. Some students have lost a parent, grandparent or friend while participating and share their feelings with their patient pen pals. The patients live on with cancer or AIDS as their diseases become chronic. Teens graduate from high school, apply to college and write college acceptance essays about this experience. Medical and nursing students go on to become more compassionate physicians. The Firefly Project has become a repository of intergenerational dialogues full of rare insights into the meanings of life, illness and death.

I have received abundant grace through Art for Recovery and The Firefly Project. At the end of each year when the Adaptations are shared with the public, the pen pals on stage receive a standing ovation. Tears flow freely. A parent tells me her teen is now able to express fears and hopes openly and has developed great compassion for her pen pal. A medical student says the lessons he learned about kindness and courage will make a difference in how he will treat his own patients some day. A patient stands before the audience and then dies the following week. I am the privileged one. I bear witness to the beauty that is life, and I remember why I do this work.

To the patients and students who have participated in all things Art for Recovery and to all those who left their legacy in their art work and in their letters, I am forever grateful.

~ Cynthia D. Perlis

When A Firefly Patient Dies

Over the years, patients have died while participating in Firefly, some suddenly with no warning. There is no way to prepare students in these situations. Sometimes a patient becomes too ill to continue writing to his or her pen pal. This is the real meaning of The Firefly Project: giving something of oneself without expecting anything in return. When I am informed that a patient has died, I contact the parents of the student pen pal and tell them what has happened, and I go to the school and inform the student in person. I tell the student how much their letters meant to their pen pal and answer any and all questions. The students are encouraged to continue writing to their pen pal's family and let them know how much the letters have meant.

Art for Recovery has archived every letter written since 1992. When a patient dies, I am privileged to send all the letters home to the family. In one instance, a student had participated in the Firefly Project when she was 14. When she was 19, she was killed in a car accident. A few months later, I told her mother that I wanted to send her the letters her daughter had written, especially the ones about what she wanted to be when she grew up. Her mom was able to revisit her young daughter's hopes and dreams in her own handwriting. To preserve history in this way, I hold on to the letters throughout the years.

The death of a pen pal reminds us that we have no control over what happens in a lifetime. How do we make sense of this? How do we move forward? The Firefly Project, through experience, allows for a safe and healing space where students can grieve and try to understand how their relationship, if only for a brief time, affected not only their lives, but their pen pal's life as well. Hopefully, they can enter into a dialogue with friends and family about what this experience meant to them and begin the conversation about what it means to die.

Students respond differently to death. Some want to talk about it, ask questions and learn everything they can about how and why it happened. Some refuse to talk about it, or defer coming to terms with this loss. Honest conversations about illness, dying and death are rare in our culture. A major goal of The Firefly Project is to begin the discussion of these taboo subjects, to enable patients to speak freely about the problems they live with daily, to acknowledge that the life they planned will not be possible and to express the sadness that illness has taken away so much and sometimes given great gifts. The project enables young people to voice their own feelings about loss and become compassionate adults.

Perhaps by reading the words and wisdom of those who have died, we are led to a better understanding of life in all of its complexities. We are privileged to bear witness because death is inevitable. The challenge is to live fully each day. Permission was given for the use of all letter excerpts.

~ Cynthia D. Perlis

About the Letters

In this book I have included the most poignant, intimate and compelling words that are the essence of each letter.

Sometimes, a patient is no longer able to write. In this case, the student may continue writing, knowing he or she may receive nothing in return. Please note that a student also may no longer participate for various reasons. In the book you will note several letters with no partner response.

Many of the pen pals, both students and patients, have written honest, heartfelt and deeply moving statements about their experiences with daily life, school, health and loss. I created a separate chapter for some of these statements because I think they deserve to be read as individual pieces.

~ Cynthia D. Perlis

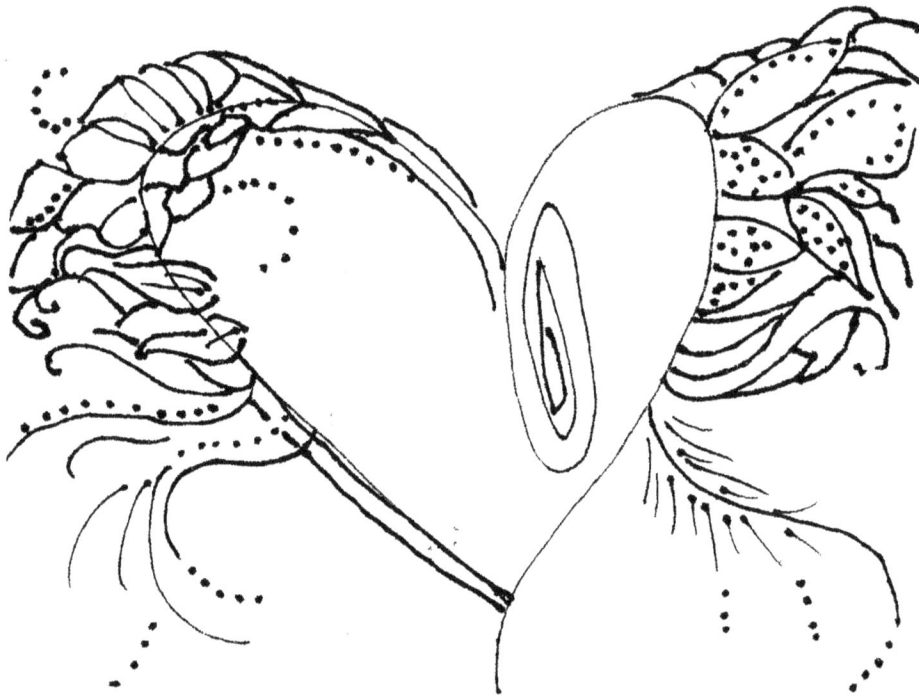

About the Adaptation

Over 100 students and patients participate each year. During the year, as the letters come into my office, I review them for content to make sure personal information is not included (emails, phone numbers, blogs, etc.). About ten years ago, as I was reading the letters, I realized that these stories needed to be told to a wider audience. I began analyzing them more carefully, looking for themes to which the public might relate. I realized the letters contain honest and deeply poignant stories about life and death. Wouldn't it be interesting, I thought, to write a script taking excerpts from the conversations in the letters and produce a public reading (with the actual patients and students reading their own words, script in hand) to the community?

Generally it takes about five months to write the script and get permission to use the excerpts. I contact the students and patients to make sure they are comfortable sharing private and personal information they included in their letters. Once everything is approved, the script is edited and divided into acts. All pen pals are invited to view the script beforehand and make any changes before the Adaptation takes place.

~ Cynthia D. Perlis

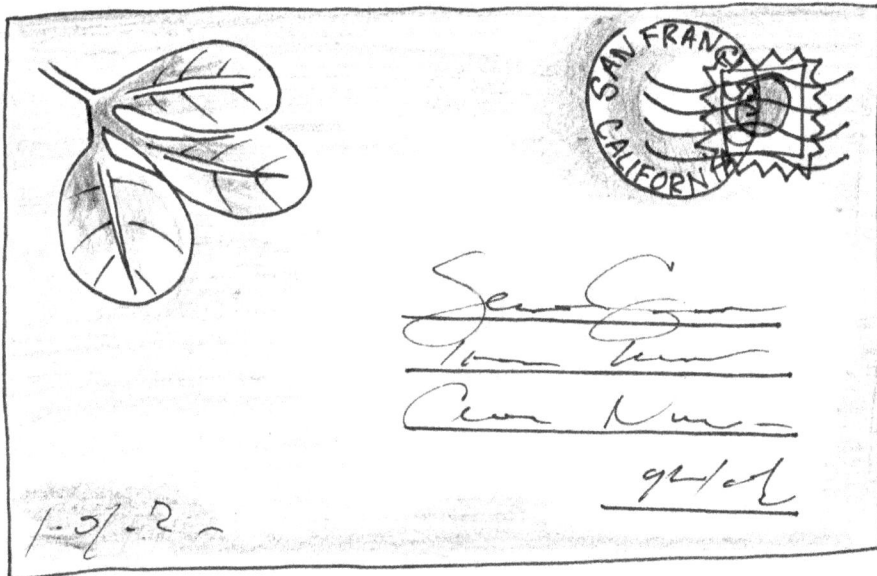

Instructions On How To Read This Book

First, take a deep breath. You will bear witness to uplifting stories and stories that will bring you to tears. You will note that some of the writing is sophisticated and creative, while some of the writing is basic and to the point. Some folks exchanged very long, thoughtful letters, while some letters, although brief, had a tremendous amount to say. You may find yourself wanting more; you may wonder what happened next. In some cases, you may identify with what is being said, or wonder why someone feels the way he or she does. In most cases you will be in awe of how complete strangers could write such deeply personal and intimate letters and come to know each other so well in such a short time.

The letters are divided into chapters. Each chapter contains excerpts from conversations which are then divided into themes. The teen letters are included in one chapter; the medical student letters are included in another. Although the Firefly Project began in 1992, this book contains the best of the letters from the past few years.

Take your time reading this book. The illustrations will give you an opportunity to reflect and think about the folks who have opened their lives to you. Know that this book is about beauty and life and hope. The adults coping with cancer have willingly shared their experiences, feelings and hope with you. They have found beauty in the every day that many of us take for granted: the moon and the stars at night, the mountains and the sea, the morning's first breath, the growth of new hair. They have found hope in the news that for right now, there is no more cancer, or no evidence of disease (NED), that a birthday is something to celebrate along with gray hair, that they have lived months or years longer than the statistics said were possible – they share hope. The students have found a friend to listen. They have given empathy and compassion freely. They know that cancer is not a death sentence but can be a chronic illness. They understand that a final exam is important, but not the end of their lives if they don't do well. They learn about priorities. They, too, find beauty and hope in life experiences; a college acceptance, a new relationship, sharing in the happiness and relief when things go well.

This book is also about honesty and sadness. Folks share their fear and anger because they have a right to, because it is honest and safe to say it out loud. What is happening to them is real, and life isn't always filled with happiness. In this book you may stop for a moment and, perhaps for the first time, understand what someone who is critically ill is feeling. You may find new ways to understand and find compassion for a friend or loved one or those going into medical professions who want to serve their patients as fully as possible.

Please use the lined paper at the end of the book to write your thoughts and feelings or write a letter to a friend and send it in the mail. Think about how it feels to go to the mailbox and look inside for a letter addressed to you!

Now, take a breath and begin reading. I promise that your life will change in some way and that you will be touched deeply by the conversations in these letters.

FIrefLy

An Unplanned Life

1

Letters exchanged between teenagers
& adults coping with life-threatening illness

2010 ~ 2011

Chapter 1
Stirred Up Like A Blender

Frankie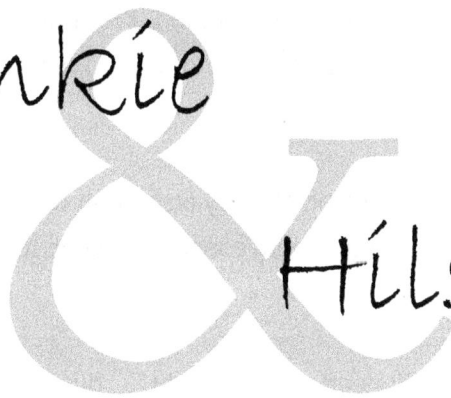Hilsia

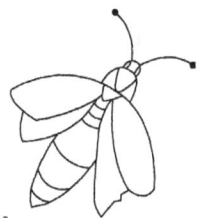

I love the water, the pool and especially the ocean. I think I was meant to be a fish. I surf, play water polo and went scuba diving. Another essential part of understanding me is that I really don't even understand myself sometimes. My biggest fear is to end up totally lost in life. I seem to be living out this year day to day, never knowing what is coming next.

If you had a time capsule, Hilsia, that I was going to open in a future generation, what three things would you put in it, and why?

~ Frankie

I have always been good at maintaining friendships; it is one of the things I am most proud of. My proudest accomplishment, however, is to be able to say that I am a cancer survivor. I was diagnosed with breast cancer in 2008. This December will be my two-year "Cancer-versary." It was a long road to get to where I am now, but I am grateful for the experience despite how difficult it was.

I see we both have a love for water. My very first job at the age of 15 was as a lifeguard. Swim instructor and synchronized swim coach were soon to follow. I guess you could say that I am a bit of a fish, too!

Time capsule questions will need more thought. . . but for starters, I would include, for future generations:

1. An Obama campaign sticker – the first black president.
2. An iPhone – it started a smart phone revolution.
3. I will have to think about number 3!

~ Hilsia

This month has been very difficult. One of my close friends was in a very serious car accident and still hasn't recovered from a coma, and my grandmother is now in hospice care in Wisconsin. Everyone keeps talking about sending and offering prayers.

Even though I continue to pray, how much does the power of prayer actually carry? Did you pray, and do you believe in the power of prayer in healing? Because I am not sure of my own answer.

~ Frankie

Many of my friends and family prayed for me, Frankie. I, too, prayed from time to time, but I can't say that praying was what cured me. At times I felt very alone and praying, I think, helped me believe that someone might be listening.

Healing comes in different forms for people, and I think it is a combination of things that helps the process. One of the most important aspects to healing your body is having a positive attitude and believing you have the strength and willpower to help the process. The alternative was not an option for me. Now, don't get me wrong, I had moments of mini meltdowns. But the mind is very powerful and can be used to your advantage.

I am very sorry to hear about your friend and grandmother. I hope both are doing better.

~ Hilsia

Sadly, my grandmother did pass away. Strangely, I feel that prayer helped me in the recovery, and processing now. My friend who was in the car accident is recovering quickly; she has even gotten herself back on Facebook.

~ Frankie

I am not very religious, but I do believe in some higher power and that prayer can be very helpful. I find myself doing it more recently. On March 7th I found out my cancer returned and has metastasized to my brain, five tumors in all.

The last two weeks have been as if I am strapped to a bullet train, hanging on for the ride. This week is better than the last as I am more in tune with my reality. I started whole-brain radiation and am almost finished with the treatments.

I will live vicariously through you, and picture you and your friend riding those wonderful waves, the sun glistening, wind blowing, smell of the salt air and a feeling of contentment.

My boyfriend and I visited Ocean Beach the other weekend. It was impromptu. We needed a little peace with the recent news so we grabbed a blanket, hopped in his jeep, planted ourselves on the sand and just took a nap. Honestly, it was perfect.

~ Hilsia

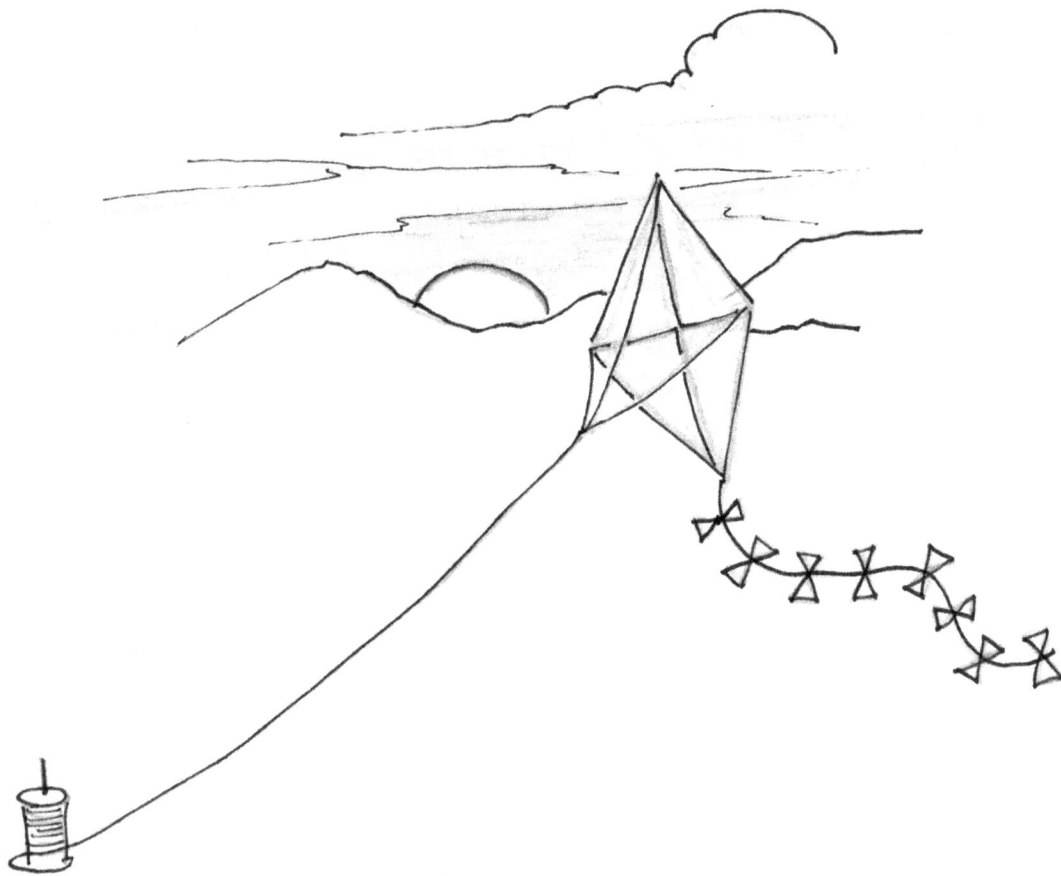

Shira & Hilsia

My mom was born and raised in Ireland, where she shared one room and two beds with all ten of her brother and sisters – and I thought it was bad sharing a room with my 19-year-old sister!

My father was born and raised in Israel. I recently got a letter from the Israeli Military asking me to join, and I was seriously considering it. My dad did it, and he said it was a life-changing experience. But then, I think, it is SO far away! What would you do?

I was wondering if you felt comfortable sharing your illness with me? If it helps, I kind of know what it is like to be sick. My aunt was diagnosed with cancer after three years of the doctors missing it.

During the summer, we didn't go anywhere so that we could spend lots of time with her. It was horrible! Seeing her in so much pain was heartbreaking. I would cry myself to sleep at night. When she passed away, I was upset, of course, yet I knew she wasn't in pain anymore.

I know my mom hasn't forgiven God. I see it in her eyes; she misses her sister a lot.

~ Shira

Your decision to join the military, or not, is a big one. The last thing you want to do is look back on your life 20 years from now, wishing you had done something you had the opportunity to do – and didn't do it.

Everyone handles tragedy in different ways, and I am sorry to hear your mom is still dealing with your aunt's death. As difficult as it is to go through cancer first-hand, I realize it can be just as difficult for loved ones as well.

This disease does not discriminate. Too many people die before their time. My cancer was aggressive, and there was no time to waste, so I quickly decided to focus on getting better and taking the best course of action for me.

~ Hilsia

How old were you when you found out you had cancer? Cancer is horrible, but especially when someone is diagnosed young. It seems as though everyone around me has something, but I guess that is life. It is unpredictable.

~ Shira

I was 37 when I was diagnosed. It was quite a shock, and there are certain things I have changed since then. For my body: I changed my diet. For my mind: I changed my attitude. I am less obsessive and critical about things, other people and myself.

For my heart and overall well-being, it is gratitude: being grateful for the people in my life who have helped me through this journey; being proud of myself for enduring what I did; knowing that my "new normal," is just as good as it was.

~ Hilsia

I especially love the fact that you talk with other cancer patients and let them know what it is like. People always feel better knowing someone cares and knowing that you can survive.

~ Shira

Sorry to report to you that my cancer has returned. Once again I am reminded that life is precious, and I have to do my best to live in the moment. There are good days and some not so great, but that is life, right? Take it day by day. Alright, I am starting to sound like a Hallmark greeting card!

~ Hilsia

I am in shock, Hilsia, about your cancer returning and I can only imagine what you are going through. I honestly don't know what to say, but I want you to know that if you ever need anything, I am here for you.

~ Shira

I can understand how my last letter came across as a shock; my apologies. I am doing better, and radiation thus far has reduced or diffused my tumors.

It is still a long road ahead, but I am hopeful that things will continue to move in the right direction. Since this is the end of our literary journey, it has been a pleasure getting to know you.

~ Hilsia

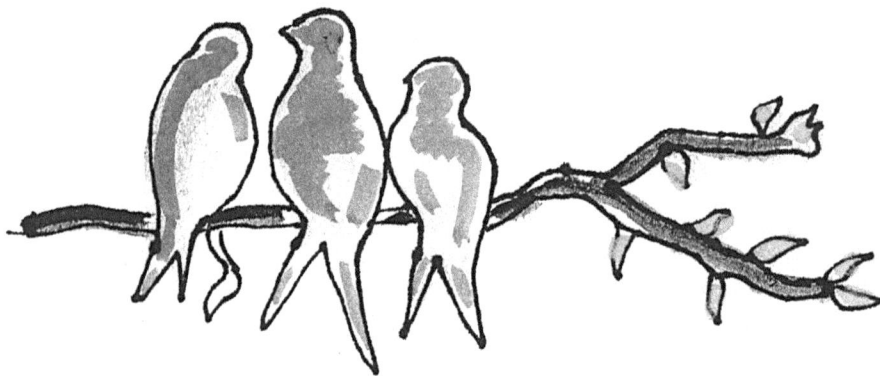

Hilsia passed away a few weeks after writing her final letters to her pen pals, Frankie and Shira.

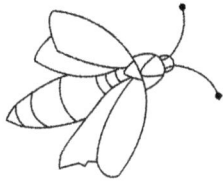

Cassidy 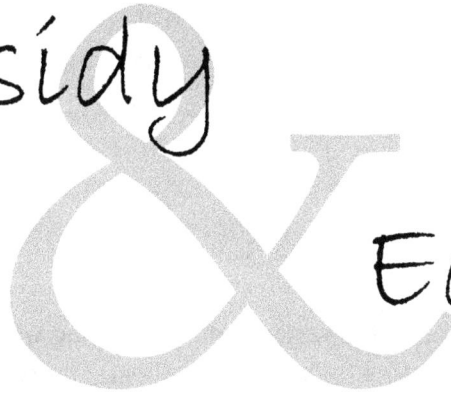 Ed

Aside from two dogs that constantly bark, I have two older brothers and two parents. We are religious Giants fans. We also love the New York Yankees. Actually my dog is named after a big Yankees shortstop, Derek Jeter!

My mom, dad and grandparents are all lawyers. Since you are a lawyer, I thought you might find that intriguing. In fact, my grandmother was the first female lawyer in her firm.

My family consists of huge Dead Heads. In fact, I am actually named after the Grateful Dead song, "Cassidy."

Lately I have been thinking how my stresses are so insignificant. We read a poem in English class that talked about how life is short, so we need to do what makes us happy, and we need to look at the bigger picture; we get too caught up in our everyday lives. The prospect of "doing what makes us happy and ignoring everything else" is a lovely idea, but I just don't know how realistic it is.

~ Cassidy

Your reaction to the poem and the concept of, "just doing what makes us happy, and ignoring everything else" coincides with my thoughts exactly. Does your teacher, Cassidy, think that one would be "successful" if he or she just does what makes him or her happy?

We really enjoyed our recent holidays. We got to celebrate New Year's two times: once according to the Gregorian calendar and another time according to the Asian Lunar Calendar. We must have had close to ten different dishes ranging from pork, chicken, beef and fish to vegetable dishes. I think I ate more at this family dinner than I ate at Thanksgiving!

~ Ed

I was recently in Hawaii and thought about our conversation about defining "success." My surfing instructor talked about seeing huge waves as he was driving to high school – he would pull over at the beach and that was that for the day. He graduated high school, and I am pretty sure he has never been to college.

But to the point: he was one of the happiest people I have ever met. This intrigued me to question what constitutes success. Is he successful because he has found a life-long passion and working at a job he loves, or is he not successful because he lacks higher education? I am not sure. But I think there is no "correct" definition of success.

I have never been close to anyone who has been diagnosed with cancer. I forget sometimes that we got to be pen pals because of your diagnosis, but I just enjoy writing letters and receiving them – and it doesn't always seem relevant to discuss the Cancer. But I guess it is relevant.

~ Cassidy

I am struck by your maturity in thought and expression. They belie the fact that your letters are from a person who is not quite seventeen, and here I am a septuagenarian and I can barely express myself as well.

I had a prognosis of prostate cancer about 11 years ago. At that time the gold standard treatment for prostate cancer was to remove the whole prostate. That was done. However, about five years ago, I was diagnosed with bladder cancer after two years of misdiagnosis. Unfortunately, by then the disease had established itself firmly in my whole bladder. So I had to have the bladder removed and replaced with an artificial bladder. Already, the cancer has spread into the ureters and possibly the kidneys.

After completing five rounds of chemotherapy, the CAT scan has shown that the metastases are now covering my whole liver. I will now have six months of chemotherapy.

Instead of dwelling on this period of life with a disease that I have little control over, I have been reviewing my whole life instead. In doing so, I have gained a greater appreciation of what I have and have had.

For instance, if I had not been exposed to gourmet food like escargots, I would not have learned to appreciate eating snails. I wouldn't have learned to appreciate the large and small thick color splashes that Van Gogh or Manet applied to their painting and what they are trying to convey.

I obviously feel some sadness and helplessness that I can't control my cancer, but I don't feel any anger that I have it. I accept it, but I shall do whatever I can to overcome it. Whether my efforts will be successful or not is immaterial; we've tried. That's essentially all I can do at this time. And that, along with all the blessings and wonderful experiences I have had, makes me a happy person.

~ Ed

I have seen where the wolf has slept
by the silver stream.
I can tell by the mark he left
you were in his dream.
Ah child of countless trees
Ah child of boundless seas.

What are you, what are you meant to be?
Speaks his name for you were born to me.

Born to me, Cassidy

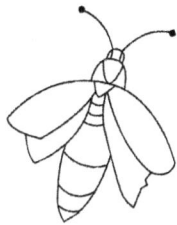

Lily & Ed

So, I heard that you do martial arts, and that is what got me interested in exchanging letters with you. I did martial arts for about nine years, and now I am a first-degree black belt.

I am currently in the 11ᵗʰ grade and school is pretty okay for me. I'm not really enjoying my time that I have to do work, but I am definitely making the best of it. I only have two more years, so I am keeping myself together. When I go to college I will definitely become more independent, and I will discover things about myself I have yet to know.

~ Lily

My martial art training helped me during my chemo treatment. Training in a martial art is intense. One meets lots of difficulties, yet to succeed and progress in the training, he or she has to overcome these difficulties with perseverance and persistence.

This mind-set, I think, has transferred over to my encounter with my cancer. That too is a formidable opponent. Having chemotherapy along with equally difficult surgeries is just another challenge that I would overcome. That has made my acceptance of cancer and all the side effects of treatment a much calmer and easier process. Now that you are a black belt in karate, don't you feel that anything you want to do, you can do and succeed?

~ Ed

My toughest challenge with my karate is knowing that I am pretty much always the smallest person in my class. I had to overcome my fear and get out of my comfort zone. Honestly, now I feel like I can overcome anything. I am mentally strong and positive and I know my karate experience has helped me so much and will continue to do so in the future.

~ Lily

Although I have a third degree black belt in judo, I have never found that I needed to use judo to defend myself. Just knowing that I could use physical force if necessary was enough to help me through any difficulty I found myself in.

~ Ed

We now have a class called College Counseling. It basically gets us prepared for our SATs. I am very nervous and overwhelmed. I just want to skip and leap into next year and not have to worry about my junior year anymore.

Man, it's been tough!

~ Lily

Taking your SAT's is like martial art: the more you practice, the more adept you become.

I changed careers three times before finally deciding on a career. I started out as a mechanical engineer. I soon found out that I enjoyed being an electrical engineer much more. So I went back to school.

Then after working successfully as an electrical engineer for ten years, I switched careers again and became an intellectual property lawyer. Again, I had to go back to school and learn more. After getting into this final career, I really thrived.

Lily, having you as a pen pal this past year has been a wonderful experience for me. I enjoy reading your letters and finding out what young people are doing nowadays. I find your letters refreshing and at the same time reminiscent of the issues that my kids had to deal with at your age. Like the SAT!!!

~ Ed

Ed passed away a few months later.

Kate & Maria Cristina

It seems crazy to me that this is my last year of high school. It seems like high school is supposed to be such a memorable part of your life; adults always talk about their high school days, and now mine are almost over.

I am starting to understand why adults say, "Oh the kids grow up so fast!

~ Kate

Your letters build a bridge for me and keep me updated. My son Miguel will be 12 years old. His voice has gotten deeper. Why am I surprised that his toys are not stuffed animals? Or Legos? It is now computer games.

I am in a computer keyboarding class these days. I have to battle my own fears about learning a new trade. My memory is weak and slow due to chemotherapy. I am not as strong, but I am optimistic since God has allowed me to live!

~ Maria Cristina

I am glad I can help you keep in touch with your new almost teenager. Speaking of growing up, I got a letter last Monday from Yale, and I got in! I can hardly believe I am going to college, and now I am going to Yale! I keep saying it over and over in my head, "Hi, I am Kate, and I go to Yale."

College is the final step before real life for me. It is like four more years and BAM – I am an adult. I will have a job, pay bills and taxes and rent. I have been so excited to move out and start my own life separate from my parents, but I have started thinking how much I like home cooked meals and clean laundry.

I like my house and my friends. Of course, talk to me tomorrow, and I will probably be itching to move out! Being a teenager seems to come with mood swings like that.

~ Kate

Kate is going to Yale – WOW! I am so happy for you. You are growing up too fast for me. It is funny how you described the mood swings of a teenager. As I was told in my 20s, we'll always be children to our parents.

I am happy to be alive another year. Every January 1st, I always remember the diagnosis of cancer and the treatment and the kindness of doctors, nurses, friends and strangers. God has prepared another year, and I am blessed to be able to live it.

~ Maria Cristina

I am always so excited when your letter arrives. It is the only mail I get besides magazines and bank statements!

I always have felt that I was gaining so much from this letter writing process, more than I could ever give back to you. Whenever it seems like I am stressed, you always have the time to listen to me.

Hearing how you have dealt with cancer and chemo and kids and moving always gives me hope when I am facing an obstacle. You help me remain optimistic.

I really do not want this letter to be goodbye, Maria Cristina. These letters have kept me sane during some of those traumatizing high school moments. I read over some of my old letters, and now my complaints seem so trivial, but you continued to listen with patience. For that I am grateful.

~ Kate

I would like to express my thanks to you for taking the time to write to me. You have completed this task with a mission of friendship.

I hope you will always remember me and the story of my life's struggle and victory over the war that is breast cancer. In turn, I will always keep you in my memories and prayers.

~ Maria Cristina

Chapter 2
The Circle of Silence

Katherine & Sharon

I am about six feet tall, so I play volleyball, a sport where my height is a definite advantage. I also love to read, drink tea on a foggy day, and to scrapbook!

I lost my grandfather to melanoma, and there is still an empty space in my life even though he died two years ago. His death is the first time I have lost someone very close to me. Death is a hard thing. How have you coped with the changes cancer made in your life?

~ Katherine

Losing my hair was the hardest. I just didn't want to part with my hair. I would wear a hat with a few strands that were left sticking out. My middle child was in her junior year of high school, and it was a very difficult time, lots of unspoken words for our entire family.

My daughter Clarissa dealt with my illness by going to my appointments and treatments. I think it was really hard for my other daughter. It was really hard for her to come home from work and see me just sitting on the couch, like part of the furniture. I was a real hands-on, controlling kind of person before my cancer. This came to an abrupt stop after my diagnosis. Our whole family went through cancer.

My mother died in 1999, and I still have an empty hole. I still miss her as much now as I did in the first few years of her passing.

~ Sharon

I hear about cancer affecting people through the media or from my mother. Your letter was the first time that I had the opportunity to internalize the effects of cancer on a family not all that different from mine. Thank you so much for sharing your experience so openly with me.

I am personally very attached to my hair and find it a large part of my identity. I can't imagine parting with it. Has your hair grown back? How has this process been emotionally?

~ Katherine

I would like to thank you from the bottom of my heart, for listening to my pain from this horrid disease. I know there is some good from this, it is just that I need some time to be able to distance myself from it. I do know that it has made me see life in a different light.

~ Sharon

I am trying to maintain a balance between academics, family, sports and my friends. As you might be able to tell, family is very important to me. With my grandfather's death, I seemed to grasp the true mortality of us all and how we are all destined to die one day. To be honest, this is one of the first times that I have written about my grandfather's passing; it feels good to express my feelings in this way.

~ Katherine

Thank you for sharing your thoughts about your Grandfather with me. It is not easy to talk to anyone about these kinds of things.

I am grateful to the Firefly Project for sending you to me. You have made such a difference in my life. I hope one day I will be able to have this kind of relationship with my youngest daughter. You two are a lot alike.

I am first generation; my parents are from China. I was born in Monterey, CA. My parents were from the old country, and I have had asthma since I was three years old. Can you imagine them struggling to express themselves in a foreign language and along with their desperation, trying to find medical care for me? I didn't learn to speak English until I went to school.

Life has been so different for me since having touched death on the sidelines. I am grateful for the days I have. I turn away from the negative environments and run to the positive. I know I can't change anyone but myself. I can, however, allow only what I want into my life. It is okay to be a little selfish and look out for myself.

I don't have to always give. I can take and not feel like I have to give something back in return. It is okay to say no. It is okay to say I want something. It is okay to do what I love and enjoy. It is okay for me to do what I want on my own, by myself. It is okay if I don't cook dinner every night. I don't love my family any less by being the person I am today.

~ Sharon

Thank you for exchanging letters with me this year. This process has allowed me to fully express and process my sadness surrounding the death of my grandfather. I have benefited tremendously from having you as my one and only pen pal.

I joined the Firefly Project as a way to get to know an individual that I might not normally get to meet. It is also a way to express myself and communicate my feelings in written form, something that I rarely have the chance to do. Something that exceeded my expectations was that I learned so much about your experience with illness and in turn learned so much about myself. I am enormously grateful to you.

~ Katherine

Did you ever tell your parents what a great job they did in raising you and instilling such good, basic values in you? When I joined Firefly, I was just looking for an outlet to let go of my frustrations and to some degree, my anger with my illness. I have shared many things with my family and friends, to the point where I felt like I was just a burden and a broken record.

Thank you, Katherine, for coming into my life and opening up your heart to me by giving me the opportunities to share my life with you. You are an incredible young lady.

~ Sharon

Rebecca
&
Kate

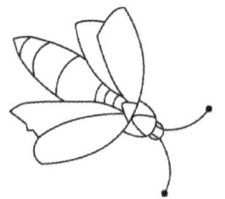

I am not someone people think of as the musical type. I am not super "artsy" or "indie" or whatever term fits. I listen to music because it reminds me of things. Some songs just put me in moods, but others bring up memories. I have made you a playlist and want to explain what a few of the songs mean to me:

The Circle Game: My mom sang us bedtime songs each night before we went to sleep, and this was one of the classics. I find time is moving too fast, and I often wish I could relive my past.

Radio Nowhere: I am in the backseat of our SUV, and my dad is driving about 80 miles per hour on the empty highway towards Tahoe. It is late and my sister and mom are asleep, and my dad is blasting this song. It smells like winter.

Vienna: I should tell myself and everyone in high school, "slow down, you crazy child/you are so ambitious for a juvenile/but if you are smart/tell me why you are so afraid." I have always been smart. I could never play sports, but academics came easily for me. And I am a perfectionist. I am getting better about that, but it is a part of me.

The Heart of Life: I like listening to this song while I am waiting for my bus after school. I sit on a brick planter and look at the sky, and I think about my day.

What I wrote you are the random memories of my life, but they mean more to me than a list of "who I am."

It seems like everyone in my family has cancer: my grandma, my uncle, my Bubby. My mom had cancer a few years ago, and a few false alarms. My aunt had both types of leukemia and is now in treatment. But despite cancer's presence, we don't talk about it much.

~ Rebecca

I loved the way you told your life in different vignettes. You have a very lyrical beauty in your writing! A little about me: I am generally a happy and optimistic person. I am also pretty driven. I graduated with degrees in computer science (to pay the bills) and music composition (for me). I have played the piano since I was ten years old.

This week has been extremely challenging for me emotionally, and I wanted to write you from a positive place about cancer. But I guess the real truth of the matter is that my life is not roses, and not telling you what it is really like for me simply perpetuates the circle of silence.

I am officially in remission. I had a double mastectomy. I have had chemotherapy and radiation. I am trying to get myself to reenter life and finish healing from the swap out surgery for the "real" implants. You spend so much energy fighting the fight that it never occurs to you to think, "what next?" There have been bright moments in this process; I have met some amazing people. But cancer itself just sucks.

~ Kate

I remember when my mom had cancer when I was in the 5th grade; she knew she would survive (or at least that is what she told us), so she presented her struggle as simply a hard time to get through, before resuming life just as it was before. But I think that is a really different mentality, and I honestly doubt it is totally true. It is more likely an act she put on, so she didn't draw me and my younger sister into her own emotions about her cancer.

I think about: How people too easily create facades and hide behind them; how the consumer world is presented deceptively; how too many of us, me too often included, live life just grazing the surface. That is something I like about this Firefly Project. This isn't some façade of who I could pretend to be – and who knows if you care about my family's Thanksgiving traditions, but they do something to define me.

~ Rebecca

This month has been absolute hell, so I don't have the things I had hoped to have done. I got hit by a major depression, and I could feel it coming. It has been a challenging process. I think all the stress together really just culminated. Plus it has been extremely frustrating to me not to work. I didn't realize until today how much I completely valued my independence and to have that be taken away for a while is a real struggle for me.

I have been going through a lot of the journals that I wrote when I was sixteen, and it has been interesting to me to discover that the times I really felt depressed were when I felt completely out of control of my fate. It is also funny being back in my parent's house as an adult. That has been a challenge too.

Seriously, Rebecca, you are awesome; thanks for being my pen pal.

~ Kate

Thank you, Kate, for being so open with me in your last letter. I don't know how to respond. In person, I would just give you a hug and stay silent, but letters don't work like that. I can't express in a letter how much it hurts me that you are going through so much.

I think it is really interesting how you said that the times you were most depressed were when you felt out of control of your fate. My high school world is all about controlling fate, and people focus on how every decision, every test, every conversation will affect what comes next. It is weird to think about fate. About how much I put into controlling everything I do and how I probably don't have much control, or any really.

I heard that you auditioned for the X-Factor. You must be an amazing singer!

There is something about our culture where people are trying and trying to get to the top schools and then the pressure – there is just too much. Sometimes, I get really excited to learn more and be successful and do everything I can do. And sometimes it just gets to be too much, and I wonder why I can't just be satisfied with a little bit less.

I have a playlist called "muse" on my iTunes that I listen to whenever I work. There is a point in one of the recordings where it sounds like someone is crying, or meowing, or laughing, or something – in the background – and it always makes me laugh!

Kate, I am curious what you feel like when they find that your cancer has come back. What you said about coming around to enjoying life instead of constantly being afraid of dying – that is powerful.

~ Rebecca

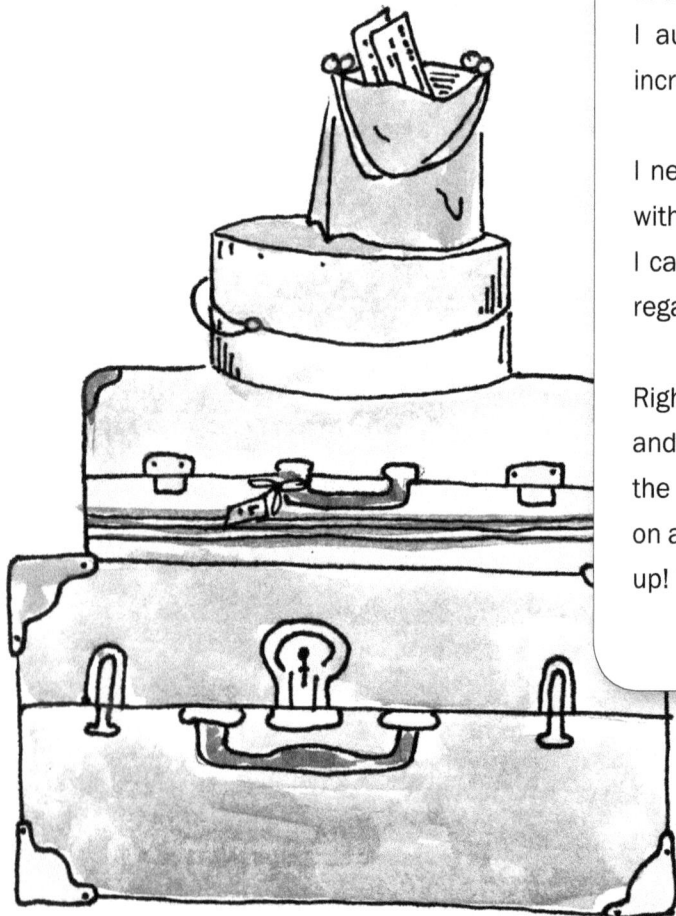

The X Factor started with 13,000 people, and I was in the final 450. So, six weeks after lung surgery, I auditioned. That's not bad. This experience increased my confidence in my singing a lot.

I need a few more months to not actively deal with cancer. I have a lot of trips planned so that I can do some of the things I really want to do regardless of this disease.

Right now things are definitely more exciting, and I am getting more optimistic with some of the new cancer treatments. I am hoping to get on a clinical trial the next time something shows up! Wish me luck!

~ Kate

Chapter 3
The New Normal

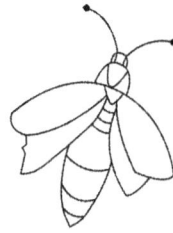

Jocelyn & Natalie

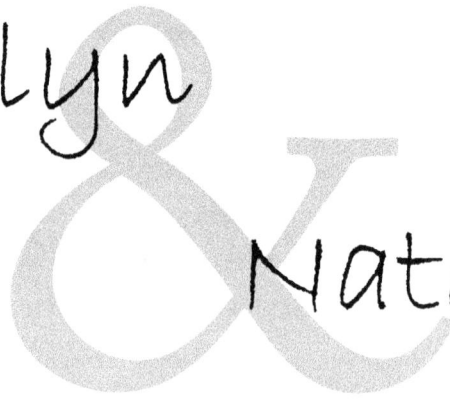

I thought participating in this project would be an opportunity to talk to someone who has or has had cancer. I thought that we had some things in common and wanted to know more. I wanted to know how it was for you to live with three cancers by the age of 31. Did they come one after another or all at once? I knew someone who had leukemia, and he died when he was 16. But for you, Natalie, it must have been difficult.

~Jocelyn

Jocelyn, let me tell you a bit about all of my experiences with cancer. One side of my refrigerator is covered with what I call Life's Milestone Markers. As I am 31 years old, and was a bridesmaid in two weddings last summer, you may expect the wedding invitations and birth announcements to far outnumber the funeral cards and obituaries – but that is not the case. Of the twenty separate announcements, more than half signify loved ones lost. Far too many of those lost are a part of what I consider my own community, young adults with cancer.

I became an unwilling member of this club at the age of 14 when I started treatment that pulled me out of school and my life for more than three months. I did not have a normal high school experience by any measure, but I managed to emerge from the lymphoma experience alive and in some ways strengthened from the life-threatening difficulties. I had managed to survive.

I did my best to move past the cancer experience by completing high school, attending college and creating a life for myself beyond cancer. I was diagnosed with a secondary cancer: a parotid tumor which was most likely caused by the treatments I received for the lymphoma. The treatment for this cancer included a surgery that paralyzed the right side of my face, and I was devastated to be dealing with another debilitating cancer yet again. This time I felt even more alone, and reached out to a young adults with cancer support group to vent with and listen to.

At 28, after being exposed to radiation I received as a teenager, the mammogram showed suspicious findings, and I was diagnosed with breast cancer. I had yet to see the ripe old age of 30. I was exhausted and almost ready to give up, but decided to fight in my own way. I continue to deal with the effects of cancer and have come to terms with the fact that I will be dealing with this horrid disease as long as I live.

~ Natalie

I can't imagine how hard it must have been for you and is probably still difficult at times. It amazes me that you stayed strong through everything that you have gone through.

Personally, I am going through some things, and it gets hard for me at times to continue on, especially when things are shaky. If it is no problem with you, I wanted to know a little more about how it is was when you found out about your first encounter with your lymphoma and how you dealt with it. I have always wanted to talk to someone who has had cancer and get to know their experience, and this Firefly Project has helped me to just that.

~ Jocelyn

Sounds like you may be going through some rough times, Jocelyn. I think high school is difficult for everyone, and my experience would have been impossible if it hadn't been for the support of my family, a few great friends and some excellent nurses and doctors. It also required that I believe in myself.

I think it is useful to write about things you don't understand. It helps to clarify your feelings – and it is the reason that I continue to participate in the Firefly Project.

~ Natalie

I feel like more pressure is on me because of the SATs coming closer and then on to college preparation. I remember my childhood as if it was just yesterday when my cousins and I would have a tea party on a small pink table.

Your experience inspires me. You are a strong woman, and you don't let anything or anyone slow you down on your long journey.

~ Jocelyn

SATs are the worst. I never understood how a standardized test could hold so much power, but it does. I am a procrastinator! A poet friend of mine says, "Everything lasts longer than you thought it would, or think it should. Everything. Except for your life!"

When people tell me that my experience with cancer inspires them, it sometimes dumbfounds me. I think that I got through my experiences by just putting one foot in front of the other and by counting on a lot of support. I did not choose cancer; it chose me.

~ Natalie

Marcia & Alexis

I guess I should start off by saying that I am having a hard time starting off this first letter to you. I think this is partly due to the question of simply where to begin in such a correspondence, but I also think it is due, largely, to the fact that I am not entirely sure who I am or how to convey myself to you.

My mom is an inspiration. She encompasses the grace of womanhood, and I sincerely hope I can someday fill her shoes when it comes to raising a family of my own. My dad is thoughtful and reasonable. He is big-hearted and a bit of a geek – so am I, though, so no judgment, and he tells terrible jokes that I wouldn't change for the world.

Other random things: I am most at peace when I am in nature, or when I am walking down a crowded city street by myself. I have always wanted to go paintballing. I am a vegetarian and I love, love, love coffee. I like making tea from ingredients in my backyard. I love eating. I think that it is okay to judge a book by its cover, as long as the judge acknowledges that any judgments passed may not be accurate and thus keeps an open mind regarding the book behind the cover.

~ Alexis

I adore large cities; for me, India is an international camping trip. I am a relaxed vegetarian; I mostly don't eat beast. I was born and raised in Honolulu. I am very digital and have all my music in iTunes on my desktop, laptop and iPod, which I keep in my car. I am very much an urbanite, and I used to rock climb. You seem focused, Alexis, clear, self-confident and self assured and mature. Are you 16 going on 26?

Last year I had a holiday in Hades. I was laid off, diagnosed with the C-word, and my father passed away. I think it would be fair to say that my life as I knew it was thrown on the charnel heap and reduced to ashes. I say this with no self-pity, bitterness or rancor; it was what it was. Was the experience overwhelming and intense?

Uh huh! Did I experience despair? Uh huh! Was I emotional as I yoyo-ed up and down? Uh huh!

As a control freak, losing control in such a definitive fashion was way outside my box and comfort zone.

Add the dimension of chemo induced confusion and disorientation to the mix and I think you have a fair picture of the abject fear I felt at times. In short, I chose to take advantage of this opportunity to change from a fear based to faith based approach to life.

~ Marcia

I should take a moment to say how cool and worldly you must be! Rock climbing, travel, music, food. Wow!

I am sincerely hoping that this year and the new one will be better than the previous. Your attitude and outlook is so admirable. I imagine you are a strong, inspirational woman. I too, am a semi-control freak at this point in my life. But to be completely honest, I can't begin to comprehend the true depth of fear/despair/turmoil experience throughout your cancer process.

Right now I am feeling like the rigor of school can be a curse as much as it is a blessing and a highly desirable education. I smiled at your mention of 16 going on 26, because my very first Firefly pen pal described me similarly as 14 going on 40. I never really felt "entitled" to my age, always feeling just too old, or just too young, until this year. 16 fits me well.

~ Alexis

I am glad to hear that 16 fits well. Age is a state of mind and I am forever 25.

Thank you for your compliment; dunno if I would go so far as to say that I am "cool and worldly." I have always been, ah, eccentric, and often ahead of the curve. Yoga and rock climbing interested me both before either activity gained popular critical mass.

Mother India lets you know in no uncertain terms who is driving the Tata bus, and it is not you. India has taught me many invaluable lessons about yielding and patience.

This trip I really got that India is my spiritual home. I traveled to Poona at the end of last year to attend medical classes, and they helped. This year, I also attended medical classes to address residual recovery issues such as compromised cognitive functioning and fatigue.

My memory is like an Etch A Sketch; the image just vanishes without a trace.

~ Marcia

I stand by my assertion that you are "cool and worldly." You suggest eccentric, another positive trait in my opinion. And I smiled at your mention of being perpetually 25. I have always thought that seemed like the ideal age.

I am a little stressed at present. There are two modes I have during the school year: staying afloat/wading and sinking/gasping for breath. I am currently afloat! And, I have to take some long overdue driving lessons. I pretty much get around on my own by bus, but the autonomy and independence a license represents is exciting and welcomed. Plus it is a tangible and recognizable rite of passage in a youth culture that otherwise seems devoid of such rites.

~ Alexis

I received your letter today, and its arrival was very timely, as I had managed to work myself into an emotional and psychological "froth." I like to use the ski analogy of the Black Diamond run to describe the feeling of fear and trepidation prior to committing to skiing a challenging run. I have experienced this on numerous occasions while ill and during recovery.

For all intents and purposes, I look fine and I sound fine; however, my brain is still scrambled. At this stage in my life, I am so grateful to be a beneficiary of the digital age. I don't know what I would do without spell check, Google and Wikipedia; these digital tools enhance my altered cognitive functioning. I love your description of the two modes you are in during the school year. Sometime I succumb to overwhelming emotions (like today) and freak/whack out. Classic kneejerk "react" versus "act" response.

~ Marcia

I am leery of dealing with death. In 2009, I lost three family members: my father and two aunts. In the fall of 2009, my Aunt Annette sent me a floral arrangement shortly after I returned from my father's memorial service, and I called to thank her for her kind generosity: that was the last time I spoke with Aunt Annette. I have not had it in me to offer my condolences to her family.

For me, I am grappling with the new "normal" and what that means. I am grateful for my health. This is Year TWO. I am grateful that I have made it this far, relatively unscathed. I have to remind myself to forge ahead with faith and not fear. My friend who has shared this journey with me often reminds me about the remarkable progress I have made: a classic example of "you can't see the forest for the trees." I am in the middle of the forest.

There is also leaving behind my past life; that's finished and yet, cognitively, I still compare my current level of functioning with past levels of functioning. There is a part of me that is impatient to be done with this "transitional" period, being in between. Yet, I know that this is what it is: *life*.

~ Marcia

My experience with loss has been minimal, I am thankful to say.

There is the friend whose father died after a sudden and unexpected cancer relapse. I felt scared for the unknown that lies ahead. There is the gradual loss of my great-grandmother to dementia. She now acts like a child and is often offensive. I am saddened by my own perception of her, and what will inevitably be my final memories of her. It makes me wonder what it is that I value in terms of life, and quality of life for me and for those I care about.

You mentioned being suspended in a "transitional" period. Though our experiences are obviously different, I, too, feel like I am in a point that lies somewhere between the stability and security of childhood and the uncertainty of the future. No place to go but forward.

I would like to end this letter by letting you know that I stand by my initial assessment of you as "cool." Not only in the sense of being hip, which you are, but in your perspectives, writing style and interests. Dynamic, lively and engaged: check, check and check!

~ Alexis

Sophie 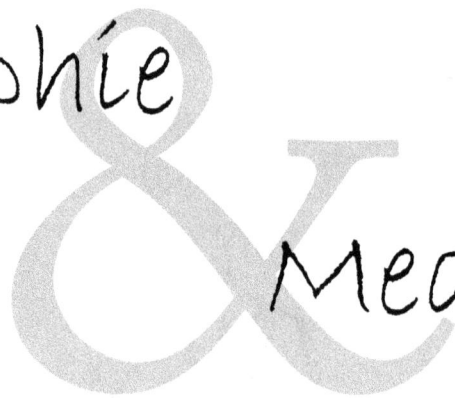 Medea

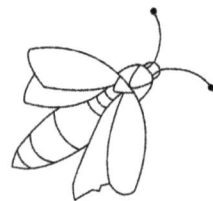

I am half Indian and half Dutch, and I have lived in San Francisco my entire life. I am happiest when I am in nature in beautiful light with people I love. I hope to be better at being a wholesome person than being good at any particular thing. I wish I could meet you in person right now, and somehow wordlessly convey to you everything I am about because I know that there is no way I will ever be able to genuinely and articulately do justice to all of the things I would like to tell you.

Lately I have been thinking a lot about the guilt that inevitably accompanies the opportunities that money allows for. I feel guilty that I have received this amazing education that should provide me with the knowledge and resources to provide similar education opportunities to those less fortunate than myself. I feel guilty that I don't deserve my blessings anymore than anyone else. I feel the impossibility of righting large scale economic disparities.

~ Sophie

You are lucky to have the brains and resources to attend such a fine school. When we don't suffer from poverty, we can use our time and our means and our intellect to make our community stronger and healthier for everyone.

~ Medea

I love my mother; I have inherited most of my disorganization, dance moves, and emotionality from her. On the other extreme, my father has the most ridiculous humor of anyone I have ever met, but I have likely adopted more of his jokes than I am willing to admit! He likes to pretend that he is an artist. When all the telephone poles were being cut down, he collected them, wanting to make totem poles. We have had 15 feet of the poles lying in our driveway for over a year!

My brother and I think in almost identical ways. We both love how strange we can be around each other!

~ Sophie

Your family sounds like a sitcom. I mean that in the most affectionate way! I can just imagine you and your mom dancing in the living room while your dad dreams up what face to carve in the telephone poles and your brother captures it all on video and uploads to YouTube with his biting but loving commentary. My dad fancied himself as an artist also. He was a lawyer but he painted black velvet pictures! He also built ship models, which explains why both my son and I love to build things. I learned needlepoint and cross stitch and crewel from my mom!

~ Medea

I have been thoroughly confused by our city's bipolar weather patterns. I have to admit that they have been quite fitting with my mind-set lately. I think there is something so grounding about San Francisco fog. It makes me feel like part of the city, instead of a moving piece within it.

I can't imagine being truly effective at anything, humanitarian or otherwise, unless I am generally happy myself. My freshman English teacher put it best when he said that no one person could possibly deserve the privilege or be worth the tuition for multiple years of private school unless he or she used their education to serve the rest of the world.

Recently I have become more aware of how often I justify indulging in pretty meaningless and self-involved pursuits by envisioning work I hope to do later on. By the same token, however, I also know that, because I have virtually no responsibilities at this point in my life, I should be taking advantage of the opportunity to make myself as happy as I possibly can in the present.

My brother and I have totally undergone a role reversal in terms of openness with one another. Although I used to be the irritating over-sharer, he's booted me out of that spot and is now the chatty one. I look forward to spending time with him even more than I do with many of my friends. Despite how cliché it sounds, I do honestly think that knowing that I am bound for college in a year has made me a lot more appreciative of time spent with my family.

~ Sophie

Life isn't fair. Lots of people have more than they deserve. Lots of smart, kind people end up as baristas or taxi drivers. I know a Yale graduate who is homeless in San Francisco. My law school boyfriend, who devoted his life to criminal defense, was just diagnosed with a brain tumor.

You have plenty of time to agonize and fret over how much or little you can do to save the world. The secret is that you start in your own circle. If you make an impact there, as you have with Firefly, then expand the circle a little. Make a goal. Be disciplined in your approach to reaching it. Move the bar higher if you need to. Be relentless.

~ Medea

My grandmother died two weeks ago, and although I have reached a point of resignation, I still feel unsettled when I imagine being in my mother's shoes at this moment. My grandmother has been the matriarchal epicenter of all family-related life as long as I can remember. Her house is the only place where our whole family gathers together. She went to nursing school and also possesses the grandmotherly healing magic, and she is the emotional caretaker as well. Her breast cancer spread to her liver – and we were told that she would at least have time to go home from the hospital to plant her flowers and to say goodbye. We were all emotionally unprepared for her sudden death.

I am sadder writing this letter than I thought I would be, Medea. I know that it would be a fact, that my grandmother would wish us to rejoice about the things we have gained from her. I oddly feel at peace, in a certain light. Death is a prolonged absence from the life of those you leave behind.

My biggest sadness comes in knowing what the loss of my grandmother means to my mother and feeling that my grandmother was not yet at peace with losing her ability to live at the time of her death. I don't really know what else to say. I know there is little I can do to affect the reality of the situation. There is no way of knowing how long we have to share our expressions of love without influence from forces we can't predict.

~ Sophie

Your beloved grandmother. I am so very sorry for your loss. Your sensitivity to your mother's pain speaks volumes about your strength of character. I know you will take the time to grieve yourself, though I am afraid I have to tell you that while time takes some of the bitterness away, it is not a perfect healer.

I think it is part of the human condition too, to vow that when a loved one dies we will never take another loved one, or life, or a single moment for granted. Then we forget the vow until we lose someone else. The trick, I have learned from this cancer, is to make the vow part of your daily ritual.

You are a remarkable young lady, Sophie.

~ Medea

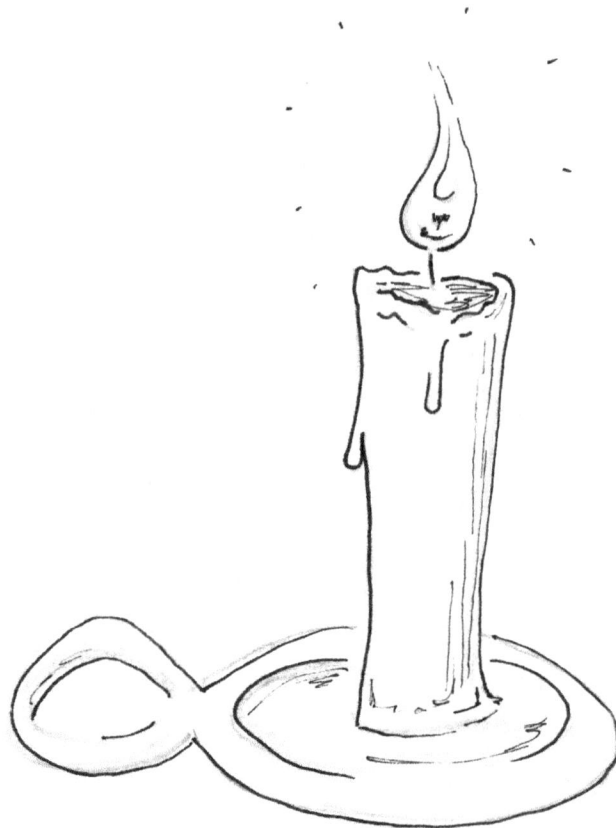

Chapter 4
Never, Never, Never Give Up

Javier & Greg

When I heard about the Firefly Project, I wanted to participate really bad. You may ask me why? I love to meet new people, I love to talk, and I love to express my ideas with someone new, some one who can understand me for who I am.

I love to think out of the box. I love to dream. I really do. I am kind of a loud person, and I use my voice a lot. I love a good debate. My parents say I should be a lawyer. I love to laugh. I am interested in good books. I am also interested in the brain, mostly how it works and what makes us love, or be sad. I am a big emotional guy, Greg. And I value my friends.

I never was a big family guy. But recently family has become a bigger part of my life than I really ever thought. My parents are divorced, and my dad got remarried to a very nice woman, soon producing a child named Oscar, my half-brother. Oscar is nowhere related to me because I was adopted at three months in Guatemala. I don't really know why I was given up for adoption, but I am happy to have the parents I have now. Oscar is four years old now and I love him soooo much and I would do anything for him,

My older brother passed away when he was almost three years old from a breathing condition. After he passed and a little after adopting me is when my parents broke up. I don't want to lose anyone like that again, never!

I would like you to know something very special about me. I love the moon, I love the night sky, the stars. . . the mystery of it means A LOT to me.

So if you would do me one favor, look up at the moon and dream. As John Lennon wrote, "You may say that I am a dreamer, but I am not the only one, I hope someday you will join us, and the world, will be as one."

So this Firefly Project is about a pen pal relationship with someone who has gone through some life-changing experiences. I hear you have many stories, so please share with me.

~ Javier

I appreciate your interest and courage because where cancer has been, lots of people don't want to touch with a ten foot pole and will hightail it as far away as they can get – even relatives, I have found.

Much of my first year following diagnosis and treatment is not fully conscious to me in an objective way, although in a subjective way, I remain very much aware. When cancer strikes, some close people fade away, and new and surprising people appear in one's life.

You asked me, Javier, what was I doing at 15 in high school? I was on the debate team. My dream? To become a lawyer like my father who left home but left his books behind.

The life path of intending to be a lawyer didn't happen. I went to work and went to art schools and gave up all ambition to be a big shot. When I draw and paint, all distractions go away, and I feel free and happy. I never believed art meant fame and money. I am happy to be alone. More of a loner. Always have been, I guess. Not that I recommend going that route. I read a lot of books. People I was close to died. That is what happens when time marches on! I wanted to be an oceanographer, but there was no ocean near the Midwest, and later I was involved in a unplanned life.

~ Greg

If you wouldn't mind, what were the first thoughts you had when they told you that you had cancer? Was it about what you are going to do next? Or how will you spend your life? Or was it about family and friends? I hope you really don't mind my asking because I have always wondered if I was told that I was going to die what my first reaction would be.

I love the night sky, and to tell you the truth it disappoints me when it is all foggy, and I can't see the moon. And, just wondering why did you want to be an oceanographer?

So this is my time to end this letter. My time to ponder things a bit more.

~ Javier

The dream of oceanography came from seeing colorful deep sea pictures and reading underwater exploration adventures. At that time I had never even seen the real ocean. Some people get practical and make their adventures come true. I never went outside my imagination.

When they told me I had cancer, I had guessed it because they told me I had a brain tumor and when it turned out that the brain tumor had metastasized from the lung, it was no surprise. When I was in treatment, I fell down a few times. I got to watch a lot of action adventure video tapes over and over and over and over again.

My siblings couldn't handle the word cancer or my reality. I hope they stay healthy. Never give up your dreams, Javier! Do what you can to realize what matters in life. Soon enough we get old.

~ Greg

Life has been weird lately. My grandmother, to whom I am very close, has congestive heart failure along with dementia. So life is a little hard right now.

The beach has a certain vibe about it. I love to listen to the song "Sittin' on the Dock of the Bay" by Otis Redding when at the beach, or enjoying the smooth rocking of a boat. Great vibe!

I am sorry that your siblings didn't respond to you, Greg. But I understand that a long term cancer illness or the possibility of death is a hard subject for anyone.

~ Javier

I recently came home from Hawaii. It was the luck of the draw that I was able to go there and stay a week. See what you can of this old world without joining a military and breathe in new sights. This is your world, and you deserve to explore it. I am sorry about your grandma. Light can come out of the clouds.

~ Greg

I hope all the troubles you have improve, and I hope that the good in your life only gets better. I am happy we are pen pals!

~Javier

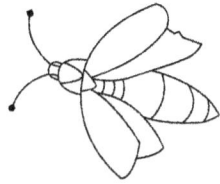

Anastasia & Richard

I am a senior in high school with some big dreams and an optimistic view of this wonderful world we live in.

I think that our past sculpts us into the person we are today, so I will try to explain a little bit about who I am.

I came from Ukraine when I was eleven years old. My dual culture life has allowed me to "live between the lines." I speak three different languages. My biggest dream is to study in Paris, but I have to learn French first!

~ Anastasia

Such journeys you have seen at such a young age, Anastasia. And to be from Ukraine, you must be very proud. I admire your ambition to study in Paris. I know Paris as I made my living as an art dealer for almost 30 years before my medical situation demanded all my attention.

I apologize if this letter reaches you late; the delay is entirely due to my chemotherapy regimen. I have to tell you, the cure is almost as tough as the disease.

My three sons have been very active in fighting my pancreatic cancer by participating in fund-raising events. It touches me to see my children be so giving.

~ Richard

I understand that your schedule must be tight concerning your disease. My letter is running late too because the holidays are always such a stressful time.

I had an urgent trip to Ukraine because my father was sick. I got to see him and help him out as much as I could before he passed away. It was painful to see him because I understood that he had given up on fighting for his life, and that is the one thing that should keep you going over any kind of medicine. What do you think? Once we give up on ourselves, is that the end?

~ Anastasia

I am so sorry to hear about your dad. You must miss him very much. I am so proud to have you as a pen pal. I am fighting the good fight. Three weeks a month of some really sickening chemo, and then a week free!

I just bought a silver Saab convertible with a rocket for an engine and a five speed to handle it. I find it makes me forget I have cancer at times!

~ Richard

I am very sorry to hear that three weeks of your month are spent in chemotherapy. I lost both of my grandmothers to cancer, and I cannot imagine how much strength it takes to keep your head high in your situation, but it sounds like you are doing just that!

Congratulations on the hot ride! As a 17-year-old, I am truly jealous. I am working on getting my license and hope that one day I can ride in style like you!

~ Anastasia

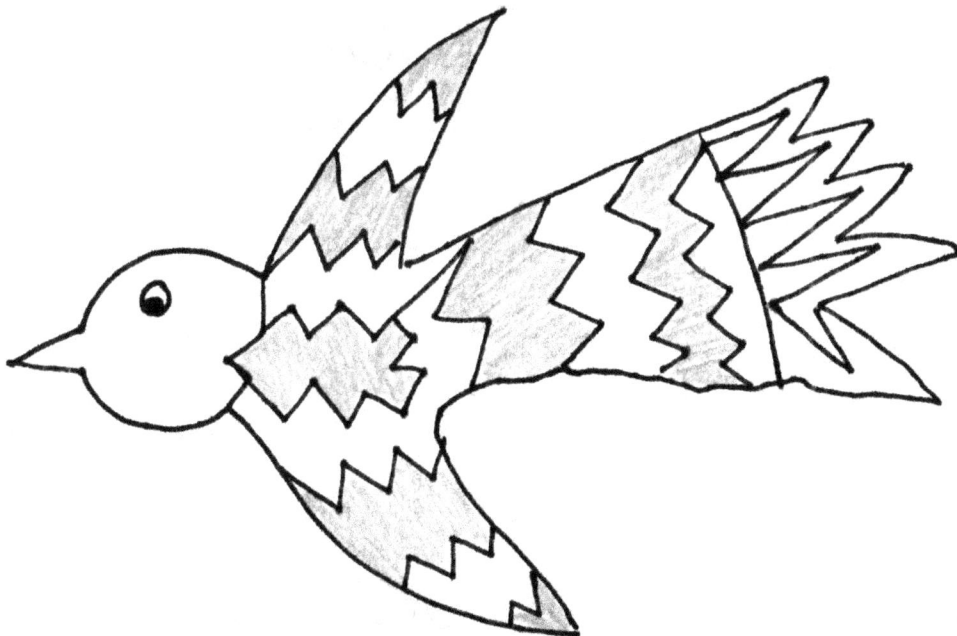

David & Richard

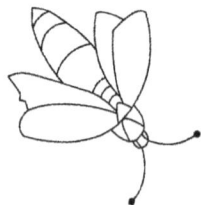

I heard that you like baseball! I play baseball at my school, and last year we went to the championship and won. We are going to try and do that again this year.

I love playing sports like basketball and mostly baseball. I really like going to Giants games with my dad, mom and brother.

I learned that you were diagnosed with liver cancer and I just wondered how all that went for you and what it was like for you when they told you that you only had three months to live. Now you are way past that.

~ David

The New Year has started off rather strange as I have just learned that I need to undergo a new regimen of chemotherapy that involves a much stronger drug. It is a real drag, but what can a person do but keep fighting, right? Chemotherapy is tough. BUT, I have seen my San Francisco win the WORLD SERIES. Our Giants! I played baseball through my second year of college. I was tall and fast, and now I am just simply tall!

~ Richard

I am having a great time replying to your letters. It is really fun, and I can't wait to meet you!

I am really sorry to hear that you have to go through more chemotherapy. I hope you don't need stronger drugs forever. But you can just get through it as fast as you can so you don't need to go through it anymore. Just keep your head up and not let it get to you.

I did much better on my finals than I have done in past years, but it was still not as good as I would have liked. Right now I am kind of stressed because I am on the baseball team, and they have to check the grades of each player at mid-quarter; that is today!

~ David

I am a little foggy on the amount of homework I had because I seldom did any. I did well on the subjects I liked and sort of disregarded the rest until report card day. On those quarterly occasions, I spent most of my time constructing elaborate excuses as to why my low grades were entirely the fault of my teachers. My mother knew better, of course, but I kept her amused! I never missed playing a ball game, though. The coach didn't check our grades.

I am sorry to hear that you are stressed, David. These should be the fun years for you. Follow your heart ,and pursue what you love. Soon, life will jam you up with car payments, and insurance and bills and all that other lovely crap.

I appreciate you asking about my health. This disease forces me often to consider the meaning of my life. That is not a bad thing. The one true good thing we have in all of us is kindness. It is a real man who acts in kindness based on moral and physical strength. Not a bad way to go about your life, I think.

~ Richard

Kindness is a very important part of our lives because it can go a long way with people. I can't wait to receive a letter back from you!

~ David

Richard & Tevin

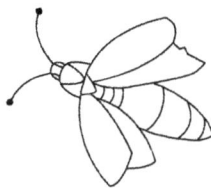

I am in the 12th grade. I enjoy playing the piano and drums and listening to music. I don't know why I love music so much, but I guess that it is just in my blood.

~ TeVin

My sons keep me up to date with music! I also love drumming. It was my instrument as a member of the school band from junior high school until I graduated from college.

~ Richard

Sometimes, Richard, I wonder what goes through the head of one with cancer? My father died of pancreatic cancer last year, but he was the type of person who easily got past things and did not dwell on bad things in life. He never spoke much about it; he just tried to live his life the best he could. How has cancer changed your life and how do you let it affect you? I imagine our relationship as being very open and honest.

~ TeVin

I was saddened to hear of your father's passing from this horrible form of cancer, TeVin. I was at an appointment with my oncologist the other day with my 21-year-old son, and the subject came up about what my life expectancy might be. I have four children and want to make sure they are prepared if things turn for the worse.

At any rate, the nurse was speaking to my son and said, "You see the difference between your dad, and you and me? We never think about our life's ending, at least not often. But with your dad, it is something he can't help but think about every day. And that IS the big difference. My mortality is on my mind constantly and affects every plan, even every purchase that I make. "How long do I have left?"

And there is no answer to that question. Nobody can even guess. So it is a big shadow at times. At other times, though, it makes me appreciate the many beautiful moments this world offers us. What a joy to live! And what a pity to become upset or angry or mad at others.

So many situations that we feel are awful problems simply shrink when you face them with the knowledge that today might be your last. Life is so fragile and such a fleeting moment of time in the grand scheme of things. I admire the way your father took his condition: stoically and so bravely silent. It is the Big Goodbye we all must face someday, and the best way to live is for the present with as much joy and love and kindness as we can summon.

~ Richard

A lot of stress has been lifted off my shoulders. I just found out that I was accepted into San Francisco State! Thank you for your words, they really help me, Richard. I believe we have many commonalities between us and will find out that we are more alike than we think.

~ TeVin

Congratulations, TeVin! I used college as a base to explore different majors. I eventually fell in love with art history, and my degree led me to a pretty successful career as an art dealer. I loved having a gallery of my own, and having to give it up because of my disease was very hard for me to do. I always have to live in the present and have plans and goals for the future; it keeps a guy going. Three years ago this month, the "experts" told me I had about three months to live. That was three years ago. So the preeminent lesson I have learned in life is to NEVER, NEVER, NEVER, NEVER GIVE UP. I highly recommend it.

~ Richard

I find myself thinking about the fact that I actually am alive, and it makes me feel privileged to be breathing this beautiful air. The simple things are truly what make me happy. I live to keep learning that life is one big lesson. The Firefly Project was a very good idea, and I am very happy that I did it. I hope I stay in contact with you, Richard, after the project, and I hope we will grow to be great friends.

~ TeVin

Richard passed away a few weeks after writing to his pen pals.

Never

Never

Never

Give

Up

Knock On Wood

2

Letters exchanged between medical, nursing and pharmacy students
& adults coping with life-threatening illness

2010 ~ 2011

Chapter 1
Humility & Grace

Alexa & Anita

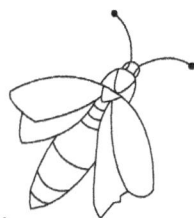

I just started working at the UCSF Breast Care Center. I am originally from Ann Arbor, and I think the only place that may be more wonderful than Northern Michigan is the Bay Area. Before I moved out here, I was told that people in San Francisco were unusually happy, but I have found that what really sets them apart is how open everyone here is.

I understand that you went to Vietnam with your husband and that the trip was really meaningful. How did it aid you in the healing process?

~ Alexa

Anita here responding to your lovely letter. Guess what? My husband Terry went to the University of Michigan. We are quite new to California, much like you. I am in the Nutrition Educator program in Bauman College. I felt that after going through breast cancer twice before, I wanted to know what I didn't learn the first two times.

I have received primary care at VA Hospitals since 2004, when my Terry received his 100% disability status due to trauma incurred in the Vietnam War.

I went through a radical mastectomy with immediate reconstruction in 2006. I have had several recurrences. I chose a macrobiotic diet and am making additional adjustments for my treatment. I am not overwhelmed; I feel ready to take additional steps to stay healthy.

I am curious about the role you play in the cancer center. I am curious how I may be of help to you in learning more about the healing process of dealing with cancer.

Your letter was received with great serendipity and joy, because a fellow Ann Arborite will be my pen pal. Today I embrace my journey as a continuously unfolding one, never ending, but always unfolding with opportunities for growth, development and richness. May we sojourn together for a bit.

~ Anita

I was fortunate in that Princeton offers its recent graduates an opportunity to engage in a year long fellowship program at UCSF. This program grants me significant exposure to clinical trial research, meaningful patient interactions, and I have not been disappointed. My job is always stimulating and the experiences will prove invaluable to my future as a physician.

How do you manage, Anita, to be so resilient in the face of so much personal adversity? Although I am still young, I was diagnosed with thyroid cancer, and I have since undergone both surgery and radioactive iodine ablation. The time that I spent off of my synthetic thyroid hormone after surgery was probably the worst part of my entire experience. Having tried to meet this challenge in the same way that I have met challenges in the past – namely by doing what needed to be done efficiently and then moving on – I have found that cancer treatment is rarely straightforward.

~ Alexa

We must acknowledge that our medical decisions will not be made with perfect knowledge. In fact, it is true of all of our endeavors: our lives are, like you said, continuously unfolding journeys. Learning to embrace the opportunities that present themselves, to transform mistakes into lessons and to recognize the limits of our own power, I believe that each of us has the potential to cultivate greater self awareness and to always refine our understanding of our own situation.

~ Anita

I am happy to know that you are navigating tumultuous personal health with great grace. Uncertainty is often the root source of our greatest anxieties. Given the time, support and the resources to understand our challenges, we learn to replace frustration, anger and unease with the calm fostered by self-actualization. As thought provoking as our letter writing relationship has been, I look forward to discussing them in person!

~ Alexa

Sharon & Frank

I am 25 and starting my second year of medical school. I took a roundabout journey to arrive at this point, and I could not be happier about coming to SF for medical school. I am not quite sure what field of medicine I might want to go into, but I have been thinking about oncology. Intellectually, my other interests lie in the brain, immunology, and infectious diseases. I suppose I will wait and see what I like when I start on the wards full-time next year.

~ Sharon

Reading what you have to say about your career, I imagine the dedication, focus, commitment it takes to transform yourself into a doctor. During my cancer treatments it helped me to focus on those caregivers I encountered. I knew that there was a good chance that my cancer would go into remission. I knew they would do a good job in treating me. Having cancer wasn't a negative experience in my life, and I sensed I was going to live. There is no evidence of disease at this point!

I have public health, and so I am grateful to each of my caretakers. So I focused on them, asked if I could photograph them when they performed services. I dealt with cancer for only a portion of my time, whereas these people chose to deal with cancer every day of their lives.

I cannot imagine the complexities of your studies. Knowing you are at UCSF, you must be really good at what you do. Brain immunology sounds like a fascinating focus. The brain is an amazing entity: complex, so many systems, chemicals, and then there is this thing called consciousness.

I moved to San Francisco in 1979, and I have seen it transformed in so many ways. My life has changed so much as a result of moving West.

~ Frank

I would love to hear more about what brought you out to San Francisco and what it was like to live in the Bay Area when HIV/AIDS was just hitting the scene. It is amazing that in such a relatively short period of time, the disease went from something that was unknown and a death sentence to a livable, chronic condition.

What an interesting way to chronicle your cancer experience. What you say about the impact that caretakers had on you is very inspiring to me and a reminder of the impact that I can have on my patients and peers.

It is incredible to me that you seemed to maintain optimism through your cancer journey. And a HUGE congratulations on being cancer free. How did the doctor share the news with you? And what was your response? I can only imagine what it must have been like to receive the news.

~ Sharon

I cannot imagine how you have the time, being a second-year medical student, to share yourself with me. Your commitment to your studies makes your caring for me and our learning about one another that much more meaningful. Thank you for wishing me well. It feels like a dream of some sort, unreal yet key to my life today. I want to keep on living with gusto. I want to continue blogging, but unlike yesterday, I don't want my whole life to be about cancer. Conscious denial at work here!

I am curating a video screening of Arts, Humanities and Culture in Space Exploration for the SF International Arts Festival, and I am working to place a rocket on the moon with a robotic rover that will do artworks on the moon. I do so many different types of work that I have actually driven myself mad to some extent, laughing at myself and this amazing life lived. I might seem to be ADD, which brings me a great sense of humility and forgiveness for the life I have created. I am working on focus and simplification, but I don't imagine that is my nature.

~ Frank

It is nice to hear about something completely different than medicine when I am absorbed in a world of people being trained to think in a similar way about all the same topics. I have been building in little "vacations" in my days where I just lie in the sunshine, read for pleasure or bike to Ocean Beach. You may think these examples seem far from a vacation, but to some of my peers, the thought of taking a whole hour or two for me during a time of high pressure is insane. I think these little escapes will be exactly what keep me sane.

Your new works sound so interesting. It is quite a cliché but I LOVE the stars. When the whole world seems absolutely chaotic, overwhelming, or I am too preoccupied with something relatively trivial, I love looking up and seeing the stars, recognizing that there is something MUCH bigger out there. No matter how many times I look up at night, I always feel awe.

~ Sharon

This is such a cool experience. I hope you can read my handwriting. Don't you love the fact that the experience of letter writing forces us to take time to reveal and read, convey and assimilate? I am loving this process, the Firefly Project and sharing the depth of each of our personal experiences.

I don't know how you do it, Sharon. I don't know how you make the time commitment. Who knows how many thousands of people you will impact? You have committed a major part of your life to self-sacrifice and fulfillment. Thank you! I can only hope that loving gratitude will be extended to you, the doctor with heart and feelings.

~ Frank

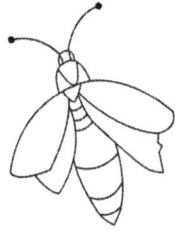

Kathy

I told my pen pal that there are no questions off limits with me – so ask away.

One of my favorite books by Bill Bryson, *A Walk in the Woods*, helped me to make my dream of hiking the Appalachian Trail come true.

Well, that and the fact that I had breast cancer. A few days after I was diagnosed with breast cancer in 2003 at the age of 31, my-ex husband sat me down and said, "Kathy, your dream is to hike the Appalachian Trail, and as soon as you are finished with your treatments and are strong enough, we will make that dream a reality." It was one of the happiest days of my life.

I am one of the lucky ones. I have no evidence of disease now. I often wonder why this happened to me. I am not sure why I believe this, but I think that I believe that it all happened for a reason. There are so many good things that have come out of the cancer diagnosis for me. I have made so many close friends through a young adult cancer support group, and I have also lost a number of friends. As a result of spending time with them as they were facing their death, I realized that I wanted to work in the end of life field. Two years ago I decided to shift my career path and work for hospice. I have never felt so at home in a profession.

I totally get the doctors who may have difficulty discussing issues around dying and death with their patients. Additionally, doctors and patients often times have an unspoken understanding about how much or little difficult news a patient really wants to hear. I can imagine that people, like my pen pal who could not be here tonight, are warned to be very, very careful about not broaching the end of life discussions unless the patient or family brings it up first.

This is a quote by Friedrich Neitzsche that my pen pal included in one of our letters and that I think is relevant to our conversations in our understanding of the human condition:

". . . to look at science through the prism of the artist, but also to look at art through the prism of life."

~ Kathy

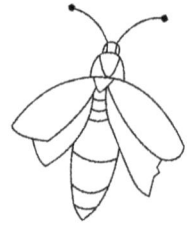

Monica & Alicia

I am in my third year of medical school. I went to UCLA, rowed crew and studied neuroscience. I was planning on medical school, but was really unsure about my motivation during my senior year of college so I joined Teach for America. I taught high school biology in the Bronx, NY, which was probably the most difficult and most important thing that I have done so far. I had heard a lot about educational disparity and was not prepared for what was really happening for some kids. The whole experience made me think a lot about health disparities as well and ultimately led me back to medical school.

~ Monica

I am impressed by your wisdom in taking time off to be sure that your motivation for medical school was something that was right for you.

I am a five plus year survivor of stage IIB breast cancer. So far, so good, though of course estrogen positive breast cancer is a crapshoot. I still have bouts of fear about it, but it is not the first thing I think of in the morning and the last thing I think of at night anymore, which is a profound blessing. It changed my life for the positive. I still live with it in a daily way because my dissertation is on therapists with breast cancer. I work in forensics, meaning that all of my clients have gotten into some sort of trouble with the law. I am spending whatever time I have left on the planet being of service. I am 51 and have been married to my favorite angel for nearly five years. He stood by my side through my illness and is my main cheerleader and support.

~ Alicia

I am curious to know what it was like to receive the diagnosis of breast cancer. How were you diagnosed? How did you process the information? Do you remember what you thought about or how the doctor told you? I had an experience where the doctor I was working with told a man he had lung cancer. I was disappointed in the way the doctor acted, sort of felt like he was pushing through the entire conversation, and I really wanted to know what the patient was thinking because he was definitely not listening to anything the doctor said.

~ Monica

Ah, the breast cancer diagnosis. That was so hard. I remember rolling over in bed and feeling the lump and thinking, oh, no, I think that this is not good. I was sent to a general surgeon despite the clear mammogram, and it was suggested that I get a punch biopsy. The doctor didn't call me for a few days, so I called one Wednesday from work. She gave me the diagnosis over the phone: "I'm sorry, you have a malignancy." I called my husband and told him I was breaking up with him, and he told me I was nuts.

I left work in a daze and drove out to the ocean. I sat and looked at the water and thought about filling my pockets with rocks and just walking into the ocean. I had surgery, four months of dose-dense chemo and six weeks of radiation. My sense of safety, trust in my body, my appearance, my career, my sexuality – you name it, nothing was the same. I got really angry. I met some amazing women in my support groups and got a lot of help along the way.

I would love to hear how medical school has been for you.

~ Alicia

I realized recently that what makes my experience in medical school difficult for me is that most of my day is spent dealing with the things that are emotionally intense. I was coming home totally drained from my medicine rotation every day, and I think it is because I had never spent so much time with people who were actively dying, and I was getting wrapped up in their stories. It is so normal in a hospital and the doctors are used to it, but I was feeling guilty for leaving every day when my patients were so sick and stuck there. Then I was continuing to think about them when I got home. I guess it is the whole combination of things that makes medical school hard!

Medical school can be very stressful. For me it is related to the hierarchy of the hospitals. We have to wait to be dismissed each day, ask for permission to do things, always let our seniors know where we are. I thought I would like this sort of accountability and team dynamic since I have been on sports teams my whole life, and I usually like the challenge of working my way to the top. But instead the system makes me feel like a child most of the time.

Hearing about your breast cancer diagnosis makes me want to become a surgeon.
I hate that you were treated that way; it is something that comes up way too often
with surgeons, that they are incredible at their craft but lack the human element
of being a doctor.

~ Monica

It makes my heart hurt a bit when you talk about how difficult it is to be a medical
student. All these idealistic people wanting to help are getting sucked into a system that
is stressful and sometimes just downright overwhelming. You have to be tough to get
through it.

I wish that more effort was spent to help doctors manage their stress, particularly in regard
to really ill or dying patients. "Getting used to it" isn't really the same as healthy coping or
integration. I think that is one area where therapists have it easier in that we are expected
to be in therapy or talk at length about our own emotional experience of working with
painful material. The trick is not to get numb or jaded or shut down or disassociated.

~ Alicia

So much has happened lately. I have decided to take a year off from school before
I start my fourth year. Somewhere along the way during these past three years I
got intimidated and felt like I was setting myself up to fail by going into plastic
surgery. I have always been interested in reconstructive surgery, particularly in
cancer patients. Actually your description of your experience really struck a chord
with me. So I am going to be working in a lab for a plastic surgeon.

One of my hang-ups with being a surgeon was that people kept telling me I would
be wasting my ability to really connect with people if I chose that route. But then
I started thinking about what brought me here and how much I had originally
wanted to be a surgeon, and I just can't let it go. It is pretty crazy and complicated
to take a year off at the last minute, but it feels like the right decision for now.

It is strange, Alicia, but your letters came at a very important time for me in my decision to decide where I wanted to go with my career. Reading about your experience as a patient helped me to remember where I started with all of this, and you provided me with some clarity in terms of where I want to go.

~ Monica

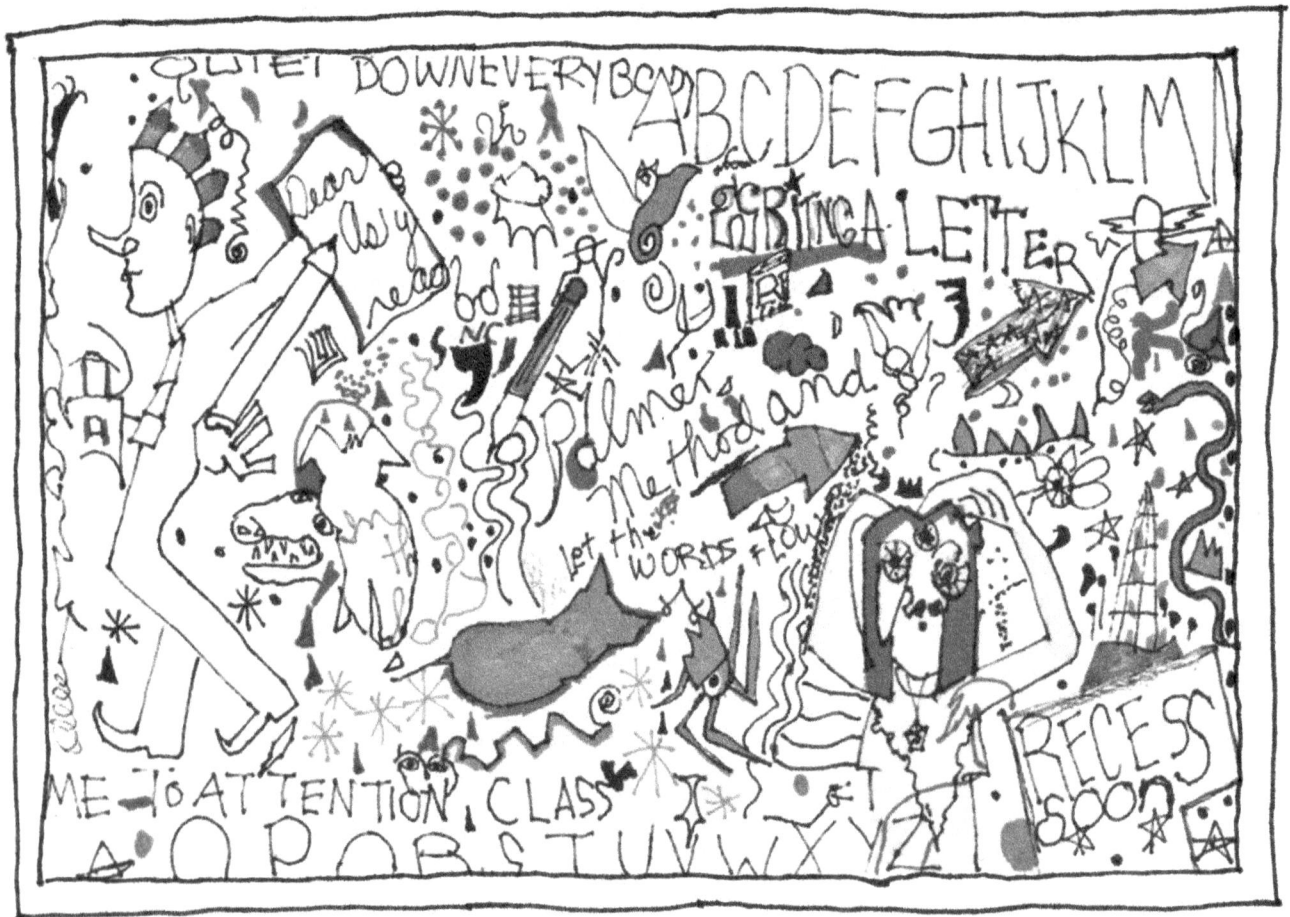

Chapter 2
Humanity & Hope

Jonathan & Desiree

I am wondering where you are and what you will be doing when you read this first letter from me. I am sitting in my room off the Castro, feeling a little under the weather, listening to some classical music and getting ready for bed as I have to get up early tomorrow for my Labor and Delivery rotation in a fertility clinic this week.

I love travel, language, art, film, culture, exercise, walking, yoga, reading and the moon. I love Qigong, tea, meditation, family, discovering new books and music, playing old records, the fall, Halloween, Día de Los Muertos and pumpkins, soup, holding hands, acupuncture and gratitude.

I was diagnosed with HIV in 2004. This was a life-altering experience for me. I felt submerged deep inside a well of shame and fear. Hiding from my family, from my friends and from the world for over two years made me feel ugly and twisted inside. The tremendous stress that I was carrying took its toll on my health.

Two years after contracting HIV in 2004, I was diagnosed with stage IV testicular cancer. I decided to move back in with my family to undergo surgery and chemotherapy. Moving back with my family and swimming through the depths of illness, loss and despair helped me to finally find the courage to swim back toward the surface.

This journey paved with tears, fears and courage led me to the Master's Entry in Nursing Program at UCSF and has given me a tremendous amount of compassion.

I look forward to connecting with you on your journey, whatever that might be.

~Jonathan

I do know what I was doing when I received your letter. It was Saturday night, and I had just gotten home. All of a sudden a firecracker went off, and then the street was full of shouts. The Giants had just won the pennant. And then, there was your letter.

I was diagnosed with breast cancer, DCIS, in June 2007. It was not very aggressive by all accounts and not life threatening. But since it was a large lesion, the standard of care was to do a mastectomy. It was simply beyond me to do it, especially since DCIS does not become even invasive, much less metastatic about 60% of the time. In October, 2010, a small section of the lesion became invasive. I finally talked my surgeon into removing just the invasive portion of the lesion.

It is an odd and frightening thing that I seem to find it harder to be a "survivor" than to be "in treatment." At my last follow up appointment, as expected, there is still a large lesion of DCIS, but the invasive component is clear. I was at once relieved and uncertain. I was done for now with my treatment. It was over. There was no fanfare. No farewells. I thought I would be elated and return confidently to my life as I had known it before my diagnosis. Sitting there all alone in the deserted lobby, I realized with piercing clarity that there was no going back.

And yet, I do not know how to go forward.

~ Desiree

I was moved and honored to get your letter. You are a talented and evocative writer, and I think that your letter arrived at the perfect moment when I needed the encouragement and inspiration that it brought.

I can recall that feeling that I had after I found out that my cancer was in remission. Here I had "won" this life and death battle, but I felt bruised and tired and strangely lacking the energy and direction to pick up and move toward the next part of my life. The moment I was pronounced in remission felt hugely anti-climactic and somewhat terrifying. Here I had spent so much energy and darkness on this chemo journey, and suddenly I was supposed to jump back into my life as if nothing had happened. I could not do it. I felt absolutely paralyzed.

I had dealt with cancer, but I still had HIV waiting for me. It felt like the monster in the closet looming large and grotesque with stigma.

I do consider myself lucky. I have had so many people in my life who have helped me and who continue to offer support and love. I consider the opportunity to share letters with you another form of healing and reflection and another reason to be grateful.

~ Jonathan

You know, Jonathan, there is such a wish in me to just write you as a "normal" person. I am sick of this cancer thing. I am sick of the undercurrent of fear and the lurking sense that there is something inherently wrong in my life. I just want to be peaceful and happy and quiet and left alone and free of all this.

The odd thing is that when I can be objective about my life, there is really nothing wrong with it. But I have a deep mistrust of my body, a fear that it just will not be reliable enough to take on any challenge. I feel oddly trapped in my own body, a stranger in a strange land, somehow not really participating in anything fully.

~ Desiree

When the body betrays, it is hard to trust in it again. I have often felt trapped by my body; in fact, sometimes I feel that I could truly soar, yet the physical is always binding me down to the earth.

You asked what it is like to walk the mazes of healthcare as both a patient and a student. I have so many complex and mixed feelings. Sometimes providers have astounded me with simple kindness. Some have really listened, treating me with compassion and most importantly, giving me hope. I have had doctors that truly look at me and those who just look at their note pad or computer. I am keenly aware of the thin veil that separates my patients and me. The border between wellness and health can be slippery and elastic, Desiree.

After a 13-hour shift as a student, I feel physically, emotionally and spiritually drained, and yet sometimes strangely uplifted by the humanity and hope. The stories that I see, that I intersect with, inspire me, frighten me, break my heart.

~Jonathan

Jonathan, the thoughts in your letter gave me a kind of courage as I again navigate cancer and everything that goes with it.

It rains. It rains. It rains. I am moving to the Sahara! Well, maybe just Arizona. There are ways in which I just love San Francisco and can't imagine ever leaving it, but my body just does not like the weather here and is not at all shy about letting me know that.

I had my year post-op tests in early March. There is a suspicious lesion on the left breast. I feel rather vindicated, though, that the lesion is in the breast that was not originally in question. So here I am with a suspicious lesion in the other breast and living proof that a mastectomy in my right breast does not guarantee you freedom from cancer.

My surgeon and Medical Scientist (my title for her) is leaving UC. I am surprised that tears well up as I write this. She is truly fascinated by her work. Sometimes she talks about her research, and she puts her hand on her chest, leans a little forward and says, "I am so excited about what is happening in DCIS right now!" I think in some ways it has buffered me from the tediousness of cancer to see through her the opportunity for understanding and the creation of knowledge. I will miss her.

It rain. It rains. It rains.

~ Desiree

I thought of you on my drive home, and I am hoping you are finding moments of sun, respite from the rain and spaces that feel larger and more open than the confines of cancer. I am sorry to hear about the suspicious and villainous lesion. I can understand refusing the mastectomy. At what point do we stop cutting away and simply say enough?

Yesterday, I was witness to a tonsillectomy and adenoidectomy of a 12-year-old boy with Cystic Fibrosis. He had received a lung transplant a few months ago, and the biopsy was a routine check. He is doing very well. The most moving part of the day came when the boy was being put under general anesthesia, and just before he fell asleep, he called out for his father and asked for a kiss; I had to turn away and wipe away a tear. I instantly was shot back to my own trip to the operating room, grabbing my Dad's hand and feeling so alone when I had to let it go at the gates of surgery.

Your letters have given me comfort too, and writing you gives me the chance to reflect on what might otherwise pass by in a blur and pick out the small flower by the side of the road.

~ Jonathan

I realize with some gratitude that it has been a year since my surgery, and I am fortunate that I have choices to make: travel, school, teaching? Not whether or not to take medication or have a procedure. I am realizing, too, that the strange, gripping force that is the cancer experience is starting to loosen, and the fact that I will never again be my pre-cancer self doesn't matter so much. It is about creating a truly generous post-cancer self, and there are moments when I am excited about that. I know the waltz is not really with cancer, but with death, and we are all in the dance. People grow old. People get sick. People die. The grace is in the living that happens in between all that.

~ Desiree

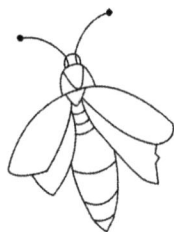

Kate

This whole experience has been a crazy one for me. At the time I was diagnosed with cancer I had recently been laid off from a job that was making me miserable. However, I have taken some time off to write music, and that part is awesome.

Right now, I am officially in remission. I had chemotherapy, a double mastectomy and then radiation. Then I had the swap out surgery for my "real" implants.

I have been trying to get myself ready to re-enter life. There is also a survivor's depression, the "I lived, now what?" which sounds weird but true. You spend so much energy fighting the fight that it never occurs to you to think "what next?"

Even though I seem to be riding the negativity train on this particular day, I am overwhelmingly lucky and grateful to be alive. At least I am alive enough to get worked up about something!

This is my first time participating in the Firefly Project. I have found myself unable to write about my cancer experience. Until now.

And I wanted to. I had a bunch of scattered journal entries, but every time I tried to sit down and write out what my experience was, I would just stop, and I really wanted to get past that.

This month has been absolute hell. I think all the stress really just culminated. Plus it has been extremely frustrating to me not to work. It has been four months of waiting for this wound to heal from complications with my reconstruction due to radiation. But it just hasn't happened, and at this point I am going to have to go back into surgery and have my implant removed which makes me extremely sad.

During this cancer process I have gotten to see who my real friends are. For some reason the stage IV diagnosis knocks down a lot of walls. At the end of my relationship with my boyfriend of five years, he told me I got cancer because I took a wrong turn in my life.

I have a scan tomorrow, and I am praying that it comes back clean. I am not ready to jump back into a round of surgeries. I feel like I am finally getting myself back from this entire experience, despite the fact that I still have cancer. I just woke up one day and realized that I wasn't dead, and I wouldn't be dead tomorrow, and I wouldn't be dead next year, so it was time to start living.

~ Kate

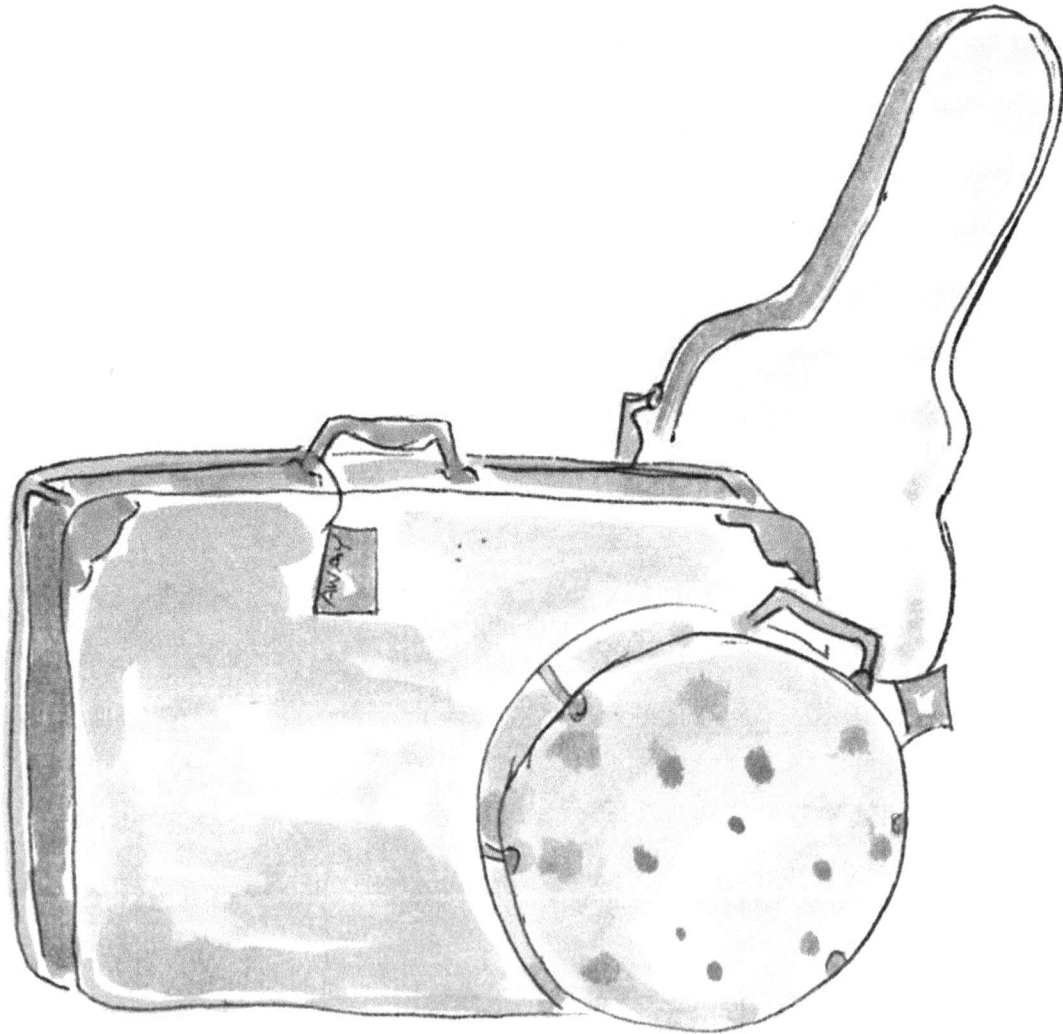

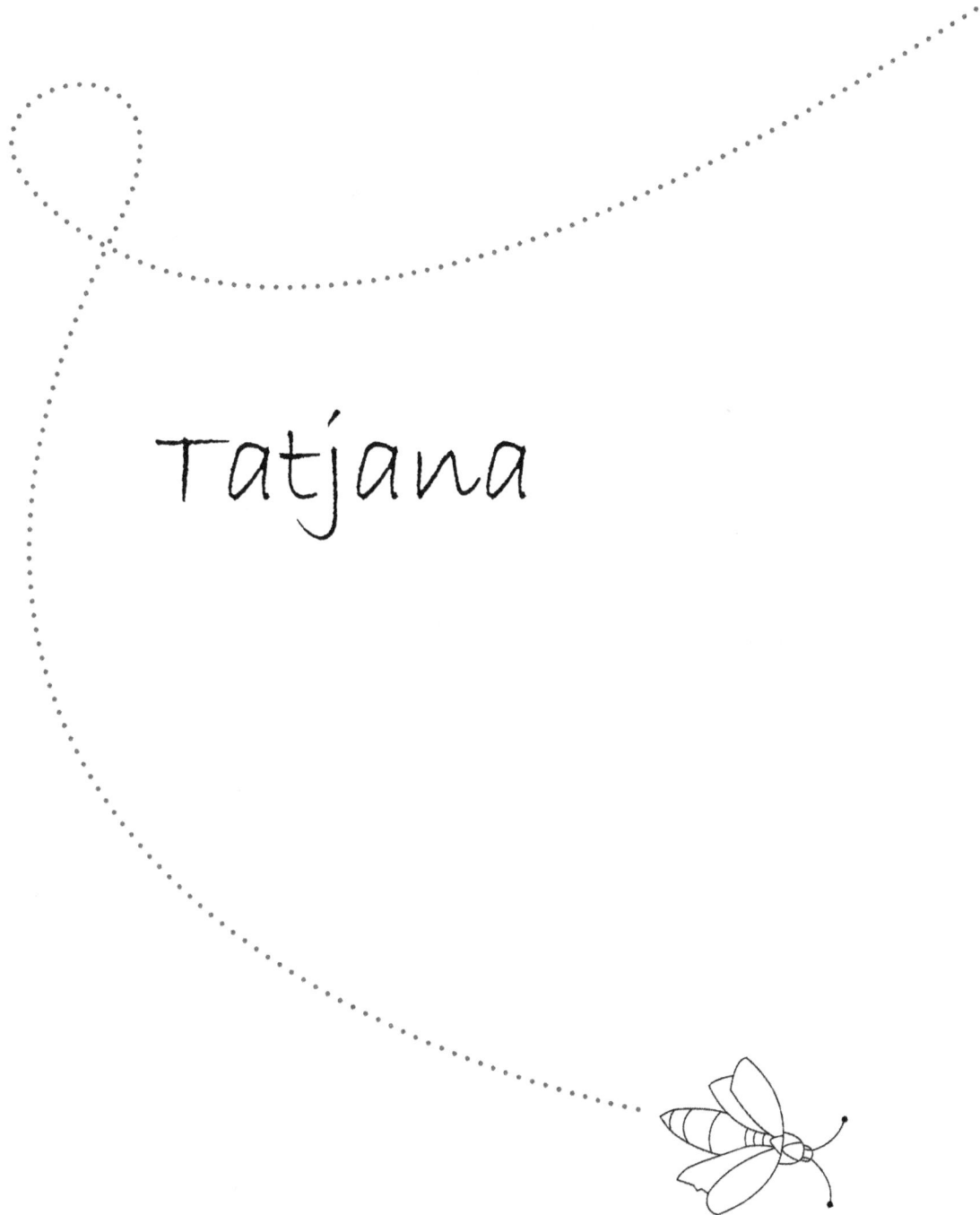

Tatjana

I never really thought about having children till I met my current husband. My desire for children started to grow in me. He wasn't ready for it, so I put the need for children on ice for a bit. But about two years ago I wanted to get more serious about it. Then I had this pain in my abdomen, and it turned out that I had ovarian cancer at a very advanced stage, and I had to have a hysterectomy. I am doing everything I can to veer the odds towards survival by working with a nutritionist who gives me supplements, a Tibetan doctor who gives me herbs, looking into seeing a foot reflexologist for immune system enhancement, acupuncture for releasing energy blockage. It empowers me to be able to take care of myself and to do something for my body. Although Western medicine has treated my particular problem, it hasn't prepared me for the life after surgery and chemo. How can I make sure the cancer is not coming back?

My parents are both working class and could never help me with preparing for an academic future, but I was able to go to college and graduated summa cum laude from UCLA. My parents taught me to be independent which, I think, helped me a lot while maneuvering through my cancer experience.

This month I have had lots of things happening in my life. My husband moved out of the house. I think it has to do with my cancer. But it doesn't matter who is right or wrong. What matters to me is that he left me when I needed him most. He failed me not only as a husband but also as a friend.

I am also very sad that I have to be alone now facing the unknown lying in front of me. Being scared of what the future brings is easier when you have someone supporting you at your side.

My last CAT scan was okay. Yeah! There were a few spots on my liver, but they have been there before, even before I had surgery. The good news is that they are getting smaller. I think the spots on my liver are smaller now because I took the liver cleaning herbs from my Tibetan doc. I am taking care of myself, and I am doing everything that does me good.

You know how people always say that cancer was the best thing that ever happened to them? Sometimes I feel that this may be true for me too. It made me look at health and my body in a very different way. I wondered about my pen pal. Did the experience of studying diseases and bodies make her more aware about the fragility of life? Did she change something in her life based on something that she learned in school?

I hope she remembers that she is dealing with humans and not diseases. Sometimes words can have more power over people than the actual disease. She said that being in medical school doesn't necessarily make you take better care of yourself – it often makes you feel guilty for not doing so!

~ Tatjana

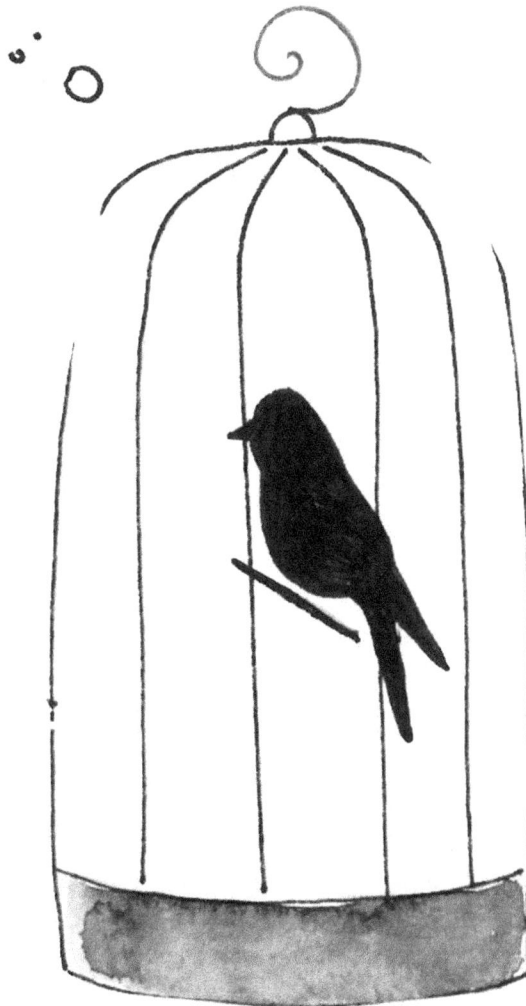

Narges

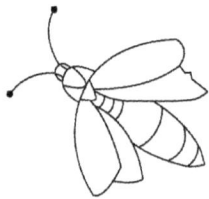

I was born and raised in Iran and moved to Orange County about ten years ago. I moved to San Francisco to start medical school and it has been a lot more stressful than I anticipated! I love painting landscapes and portraits. I have been trying to learn horseback riding, though I am not very good at it.

I was born in the last year of an eight year long war between Iran and Iraq when Tehran was being bombarded. My parents were both ex political prisoners, and they had been released only a few years before I was born. We lived in a poorer area of Tehran as they had to start from scratch. I don't remember anything about the war, but apparently every time the sirens would go off, we all had to go to the basement and lie flat on the ground.

I have two older brothers, and for the first 11 years of my life we shared a small bedroom that provided so much entertainment for us that I actually miss it. Then my brothers moved to Southern California to go to college as my parents wanted them to get a better education in the US. A couple years later my mom and I moved too. Right now my mom and dad are back in Iran. But we see them often.

At first, I was very excited about medical school because I got to meet so many new friends and motivated people, and I felt great to be part of it. I still do. But I miss giving up some things in my life that used to make it more whole and meaningful. I miss having the time to paint, or dancing.

My life has been speeding past like a bullet train lately. I can't believe that I only have a few months left of my first year of medical school. It still seems like it was last week that I got oriented to this campus and life in San Francisco. Now I am off making plans to go to Ecuador for a month over the summer. The last time I visited a country to do medical work, I got so ill I had to be flown out of the country! So it took a bit of mental effort to get myself to sign up for this trip.

~Narges

Triveni & Greg

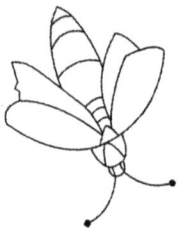

I am a second-year medical student and an always inspiring writer, artist, dancer, do-gooder, runner, yogi and much more. I am hoping that our letters, Greg, will give me time to reflect and allow me an eye into the world of someone else, particularly someone who has lots of knowledge of what it means to be a patient and the human on the other side of the medical encounter.

~ Triveni

My first year after brain surgery and radiation and chemo has foggy aspects to it, so I have gotten my best friend to remind me what happened in my little medical adventure. This December it will be five years since diagnosis and treatment. I remember poorly the objective details. I do remember aspects of it deeply: the radiation and chemo and difficulties along the way. It all started with migraine headaches of growing severity, which led to the discovery of the tumor, then learning it was cancer. I had stage IV cancer that originated in the lung and spread to my brain.

My problem was to keep from falling down: falling down stairs, falling down while crossing the street. At times the way out of a mess was the kindness of strangers.

I don't use the word "survivor" often, as I think of cancer veterans. Some people dislike that word because it means military stuff to them. I said, "Cancer is a war." There is no sweetness in it. There is no goodness in the disease. Certainly there is no romance in it. It is a viscous killer. I am grateful for my good doctors who are surprised I am still alive (knock on wood).

What defines personal sanity for me is painting on canvas and other things because when I do that, conundrums float away. Triveni, I know actual happiness when immersed in art.

~ Greg

As fate would have it, I received the package of your amazing letters, poems and drawings the night before my Hematology/Oncology exam. It was such a welcome human reminder of how my many hours of isolation in study are relevant. And how the diseases I am studying touch people and bring out creativity and honesty about life that cannot be achieved by everyone.

~ Triveni

I think I change every ten years. Some of it is growing older, some of it is growing with hunger to create. I look for latent order in the chaos. I sense the world is changing for good and bad. I think the flashy present is a new Dark Ages.

I found paintings I had put in trunks when I moved here years ago. I see I was involved in the issues of chaos even then. Some pictures can be given new life with further work.

I go to a poetry group once a month and Art for Recovery every week. Otherwise, "I Don't Get Around Much Anymore," an early 20th century song sung by a torch singer on 78 rpm records. Most of my travel is San Francisco; essentially, I have found inner travel a way to promote personal health.

I appreciate your ambition to place yourself, your life force into healing. I thank you.

~ Greg

I thought about the recent events of peaceful uprising in Egypt, when I received your letter, and thought about how it was an example of peaceful, productive chaos. And about how this ever changing, even faster changing world can be a force for the better.

I am in a rather stressful period of school and waiting to put the books away and start my clinical work with patients. Once again, your letter arrived in a magically timely way. I spent the last five weeks studying for my board exams morning until night. I was truly in a tunnel of social isolation.

Just a day before, your letter arrived in the mail. It was a little encouraging push to get me through the last of studying, and a reminder that I was working towards something human, something more than a test on paper. You encourage me more than you will ever know.

I am entering a big transition from books to patient care as I start my third year. It is terrifying and exciting to finally start doing the things that I always thought doctors do.

~ Triveni

In this stage of my life, uncontrolled cellular growth changed my present and future and led me on a path I did not consciously foresee. The long and difficult work to rub out the beast helped me to make it back to shore.

Thank you for being there, for your self-knowledge and creative work. Your embrace of your vocation is a blessing on this world.

~ Greg

The Space Between

3

Letters exchanged between teenagers
& adults coping with life-threatening illness

2011 ~ 2012

Chapter 1
The Power of Relationships

Jimmy & Karen

How was your life before cancer? What were you diagnosed with? How did it change your life?

~ Jimmy

It has been a difficult time for me. I had lobular breast cancer. It is often hard to detect on a mammogram as it grows differently than ductal. Ductal grows more like a mass, whereas lobular grows in thin sheets, and therefore, is harder to detect. I unfortunately passed this on to my daughter; my son has not yet been tested. But men can also develop breast cancer, so it will be important for him to be tested.

My great grandparents were immigrants from Romania. I inherited my cancer gene mutation from my grandmother who was from Mazatlan. It is called BRCA2 gene mutation. This mutation doesn't fix cells when they replicate so the cancer replicates itself – not a good thing. I now take a medication that stops the hormones that feed the cancer in my body. That is the theory anyway. They didn't have that when my grandmother had breast cancer.

My life has changed quite a bit since I had cancer. I stopped traveling, obviously; I miss that. I decided to join a group called Toast Masters to learn how to speak more effectively to a group. It is scary to me, but fun.

~ Karen

My favorite place that I have traveled so far would be Cambodia. I am half Cambodian. When I was in 8th grade my parents allowed me to travel there. I felt that the life style was so different, and I received a new perspective of the world.

One of the things I really like to do out of school besides skateboarding is basketball, but I am also in the CADET program. This program helps me to prepare to become a police officer in San Francisco. But I am not sure I want to become an officer, as I might want to join the Marine Corps. I feel that I should do something for my country. But I am not sure yet.

~ Jimmy

I am so excited that you were able to go to Cambodia and see a bit of your heritage. I love to learn how other people live. I also think it is interesting how other cultures perceive the world.

What do your parents think about you joining the military? My work with the military was interesting and rewarding, but the families are separated from friends and their own families so frequently. The military provides some great opportunities, and many challenges.

~ Karen

My parents are really supportive in what I want to be when I grow up. They don't mind if I go to the military as long as I have a stable income to help support myself.

My parents were five years old when they came to the US, so they became very Americanized. I know some things from my culture from my grandparents, but not that much. I am really close to my dad. He talks to me the most about everything. He is a very wise person, and most of the advice I get is from him.

~ Jimmy

It is important and interesting, I think, Jimmy, to know the history of your family. I am glad your family enjoys spending time together, and they are supportive of whatever you want to be. We can have all the money in the world, but if we don't have people to love, it is not worth much. At least that is how I feel.

~ Karen

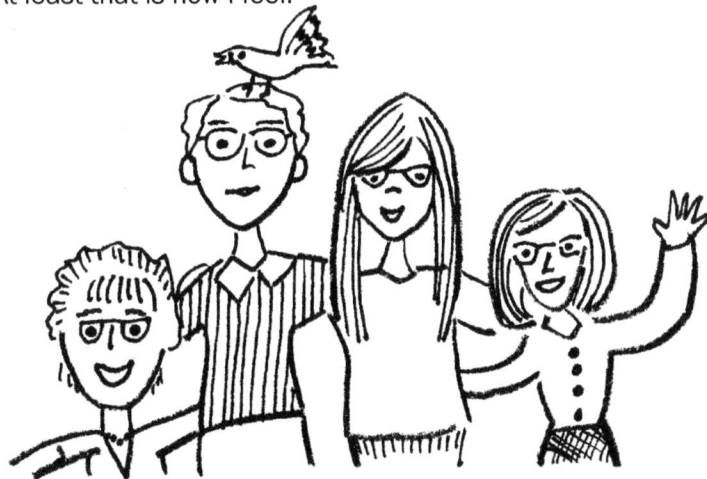

Maddy & Nanci

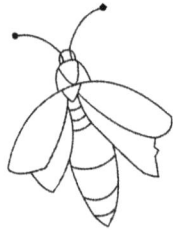

I love volleyball so much, especially because my coach this year is so inspiring. I like to hang out with my family, read, play and listen to music and hang out with my friends. I really like high school so far, but it is A LOT of work.

~ Maddy

I don't know much about new music. I tend to listen to music like Tibetan monks chanting. I listen to this music during acupuncture where I feel no pain, no body, and no world. It is like heaven.

So about me. Well, life was going along nice and easy, and I was in good health. My greatest fear, however, was that I or somebody close to me would have brain surgery. I had this fear for years. Well, I had to learn to face my fears. Three of my friends have had brain cancer! Then there was me. In February of 2006, I found out that I had an arterial venus malformation. So I had to have brain surgery! I had very little deficit, but I did have some. Then, in 2008 I was diagnosed with endometrial cancer.

I had surgery, 12 weeks of chemo and then 28 weeks of radiation. They didn't tell me that chemo brain is like dementia. I used to inhale books. Now every time I start to read I just get sleepy. I just pray someday that it will go away.

~ Nanci

It sounds like you have had many experiences with cancer that really affected your life. It seems very hard. I am not sure I can say I know how you feel because I definitely haven't experienced cancer on the level you have.

About me: I am not sure what I would like to be when I grow up. Maybe something with little kids because I love playing with them.

I am jealous of your artistic ability. I always think my art is bad. I think dreaming is really important, though. If you don't dream, you never go anywhere. I like dreams, because they take me away from the hustle and bustle of reality. What super power would you want if you had one wish? I would want to fly!

~ Maddy

I used to have fabulous feature-length dreams that when I was feeling really depressed, I would get a fabulous dream that was affirming of me and my art work. What would I wish for? A Utopian society. No money. Everything is free. Everybody has a job. Everyone loves everybody. But that isn't happening anytime soon.

Do you have any fears, Maddy?

~ Nanci

I have always known about people having cancer, Nanci, but I have never really known much beyond the fact that it is a sickness. It sounds so hard and like a continuous fight. I want to say "I'm sorry" but I feel like that doesn't cut it. People say we are put on the Earth for some reason, but I haven't quite figured out mine yet. Have you?

Hmm, yeah I have fears. The big ones are BUGS (ew!). They scare me to death, and I fear losing people close to me. And getting into a plane crash. Pain mostly. I am scared of the process of dying, but I am not actually afraid of dying. It is more like I am not scared of being gone, because I will miss the happy times I had in my life.

~ Maddy

You mentioned pain. Well, you would be surprised how much you can handle. When I do art, I tend to forget the pain. You mentioned being afraid of bugs. Well, in many cases bugs are your friends, and if you get stuck in the wilderness, you can turn over some rocks and eat the bugs. That is what they teach in the Marines.

Take care, Maddy, and have a good life. Try new things. Work for free. Do things that don't compute. Love one another. Be brave. Cry; it feels good. Laugh a lot. Watch funny movies. Make up stupid jokes. Keep an open mind. I know now that our pen pal project is over we will part ways, but we will have great memories!

~ Nanci

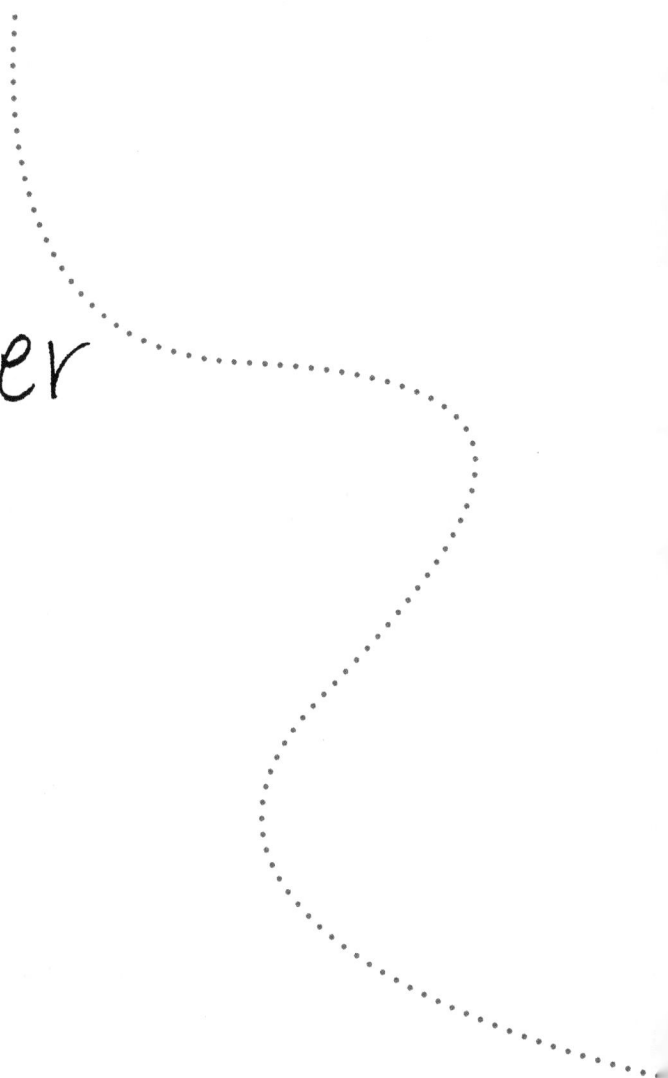

Javier

My pen pal, Jonathan, just had surgery last week, and he didn't feel well enough to be here tonight. He was a limousine driver to Hollywood celebrities, until he retired because of his diagnosis. He drove the celebrities to the Emmy, Grammy and Oscar Awards. He said that my parents would know some of the people he drove to dinner after her TV tapings. One was Dinah Shore!

Wow, a private limousine driver for celebrities! Wow! What was that like, I wondered? You know, I always wanted to ride in a limousine, and I haven't yet, but my friends and I are thinking about pooling money for the prom to rent one.

I am a huge social guy. I love to talk, have a good time and help my friends. I love my friends, and they are my life. I love to help people, and I think it is caused by basically growing up in a runaway homeless youth Shelter because my mom is the CEO of one located in California. So I know the ins and outs of therapy and the system of social justice.

I would like to be a forensic psychologist, which is all about criminals. And I am interested in law. I guess this is a whole lot of mumbo jumbo but that is kind of how I am.

This is what I love: the sunset, and the moon and the stars! The city. The sky at night. I really love the night! The moon and the stars; it really quite amazes me how the moon can control our tides and light up the dark night with all the beautiful constellations and the history behind them.

Jonathan was diagnosed with prostate cancer. The radiation caused great damage to his bladder, and he lives with severe pain daily. He said only when he is asleep is he out of pain. I feel so bad for him.

By the way this is my second year doing Firefly. Writing letters back and forth is a lot more rewarding than emails, text messages, calls or any other form of the new technology we have these days. And it is cool!

I absolutely love the photographs that Jonathan sent me. He is quite the photographer. The picture of the Coca Cola light-up billboard is pretty awesome. I decided to send him photographs that I have taken. One is called "alphabet art". Alphabet art is words made of photos. The one I sent him is of his name, and each of the letters was taken here in the beautiful city of San Francisco.

In school we are learning about the immigration of our own families, and I am an immigrant as well. I don't know much about my immigration from Guatemala, but I recently found out who my birth parents are! Not what they look like, just their names, and I also found out I have eight brothers and sisters, but only three brothers are documented. It is wild. Realizing I have 8 other people out there with my DNA or partial DNA is exciting and shocking news, and my school helped me to figure all this out! Jonathan told me that he has no family and instead of being adopted, he was put in a foster home. I wondered why he doesn't know who his biological parents are? He said his legal guardian was a Superior Court Judge in Los Angeles, but when he turned 18, he was on his own. He could have eight brothers and sisters somewhere too, like me.

I love how positive my pen pal is, in spite of his pain. I have recently felt that I am becoming a bit like that. Or else, I hope I am. I guess we all have to live with some physical pain, some more than others. Which sucks, but I guess we live and move on. Or learn to deal with it?

I have been trying to balance everything: family, school, the play I am in, and friends, but is has been very chaotic. I like it, but then again I don't get much sleep. It is 2:15 am, and I am just finishing up on a lot of loose ends; school work, laundry and this letter. I am listening to Burt Bacharach: "What the world needs now is love." My pen pal likes Burt Bacharach too.

I wanted to let Jonathan know that I hope his pain goes away, I hope he keeps taking photographs, and I want to let him know that things are good and right now in my life, calm and settled. I want him to remember: what the world needs now is love.

~ Javier

Shirley & Brenda

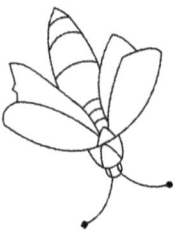

I love food, and my habits have improved with cancer: limiting grease, and being more mindful about antioxidants. I am very grateful of my cancer prognosis. I tolerated the chemo pretty well. I work at the information desk at Mount Zion. It is ironic to be assisting patients with cancer and then to acquire cancer. I have seen a lot of hope and triumph and said goodbye to many warriors. Therefore, my work experience gave me a sense of what was ahead.

This year has been a triple whammy: menopause, turned fifty and diagnosed with cancer: a slow growth, stage I tumor on my thymus gland, above my heart.

I have non-Hodgkin's lymphoma in the media sternum. I tolerated the chemo with the help of Benadryl, ginger ale and yogurt.

I have a dog, Moo Moo, and then I got Buster. My former witty boss nicknamed them Bustamoo!

~ Shirley

I am so happy you are an animal lover. It is true that animals sense certain things that humans can't, which is one of the reasons I love them so much.

I have danced Flamenco for about six years now. You would think that since my mom is from Spain she would have introduced me to Flamenco, but a soccer friend actually told me about a program. The average age of the dancers is about 50 plus years of age, but Rosie is 80 and is one of the fastest learners in the class.

I am happy to hear your cancer is treatable! I am sorry you had to go through so much. Wow, I can't imagine what it must feel like to go through six months of chemotherapy.

~ Brenda

Great news, the tumor has shrunk 90%! Flamenco and soccer: what a wonderful combination. Your interests are a beautiful blend of renaissance. You are an old soul.

~ Shirley

Yay! I am so happy for your amazing progress. The picture in my mind of a curvy middle-aged horse plowing through a field for six months made me think about cancer in a whole different way. Never in a million years would I have thought that the spiritual and mental pain of going through cancer would be just as bad or worse than the physical pain. I don't know if I could go through the battle that you had to endure – correction – I wouldn't be able to without having some mental breakdown; so for that I salute you.

Shirley, I don't always make good choices, but picking you as my pen pal was undeniably a great choice.

~ Brenda

Initially the doctor predicted my regimen would have been finished by March. My blood panel, specifically the white cells, the warriors that fight off infection, have been running extremely low. When they reach a certain level, I can start phase two: radiation. The cancer journey is so individual.

I thank you for choosing me as your pen pal. Your questions and thoughtfulness forced me to process and organize the chaos from the treatment of cancer. I am so happy to be meeting you. I just returned from Hawaii, and I am buzzed from sunshine.

I leave you with this from the song, "Mr. Know It All" by Kelly Clarkson from my playlist to shake off cancer: "Think you know me? You don't know a thing about me. You don't have the right to tell me where to go. Trying to bring me down I ain't going down. I'm living my truth without your lie. Mr. Know It All – you don't know a thing about me."

~ Shirley

Luz

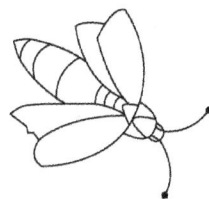

My pen pal asked me, "What do you love?" I love my son, seven years old, with teeth in all kinds of stages of falling out and growing back in; I love his long lashes and the fact that he is a total airhead who loves dancing to the song Dynamite. I love several people, and I love them a lot, but having a son is the most singular thing I have ever done, and my love and connection to him is unlike anything else.

I love beauty and goodness. I love anything Bach. I love the beauty of words. The inventiveness and ingenuity of the human mind never ceases to amaze me. The ability to: posit a theory, to create a poem, a plot, a theorem; to build a bridge, to draw a map from a walk across the land; those feats move me to the core. I love generosity. I love voluntary sharing. I love the spontaneous consideration of others when deciding which course of action to take. I love when someone does not equate absence of wrongdoing with goodness. I love empathy. For all this "love talking" I believe in conflict as a fundamental element of the human condition.

In the same way that I love a lot, I would say that I also can dislike intensely. I have a quick tongue and enough of an aggressive instinct that I can say things that I regret having said after I cool down.

Most of the people I knew when I was in my teens and who were my age, bored me to tears, I kid you not. Over time, however, people have surprised me a lot, and overwhelmingly in a good way. I have been amazed by unexpected acts of tolerance and generosity towards myself and others.

My high school pen pal could not be here, but I am moved by my pen pal's unadulterated passion and, from the very depths of myself, I hope that she doesn't become jaded and pursues every single thing that makes her tick.

I wish my son will be like my pen pal when he is older. Life is a contact sport; it is to be lived, touched, smelled, heard, felt. Be free to fly, be free to take calculated risks and make mistakes, and be free to commit – that is also a way of exercising freedom.

~ Luz

Chapter 2

Nothing Changes
But Everything Changes

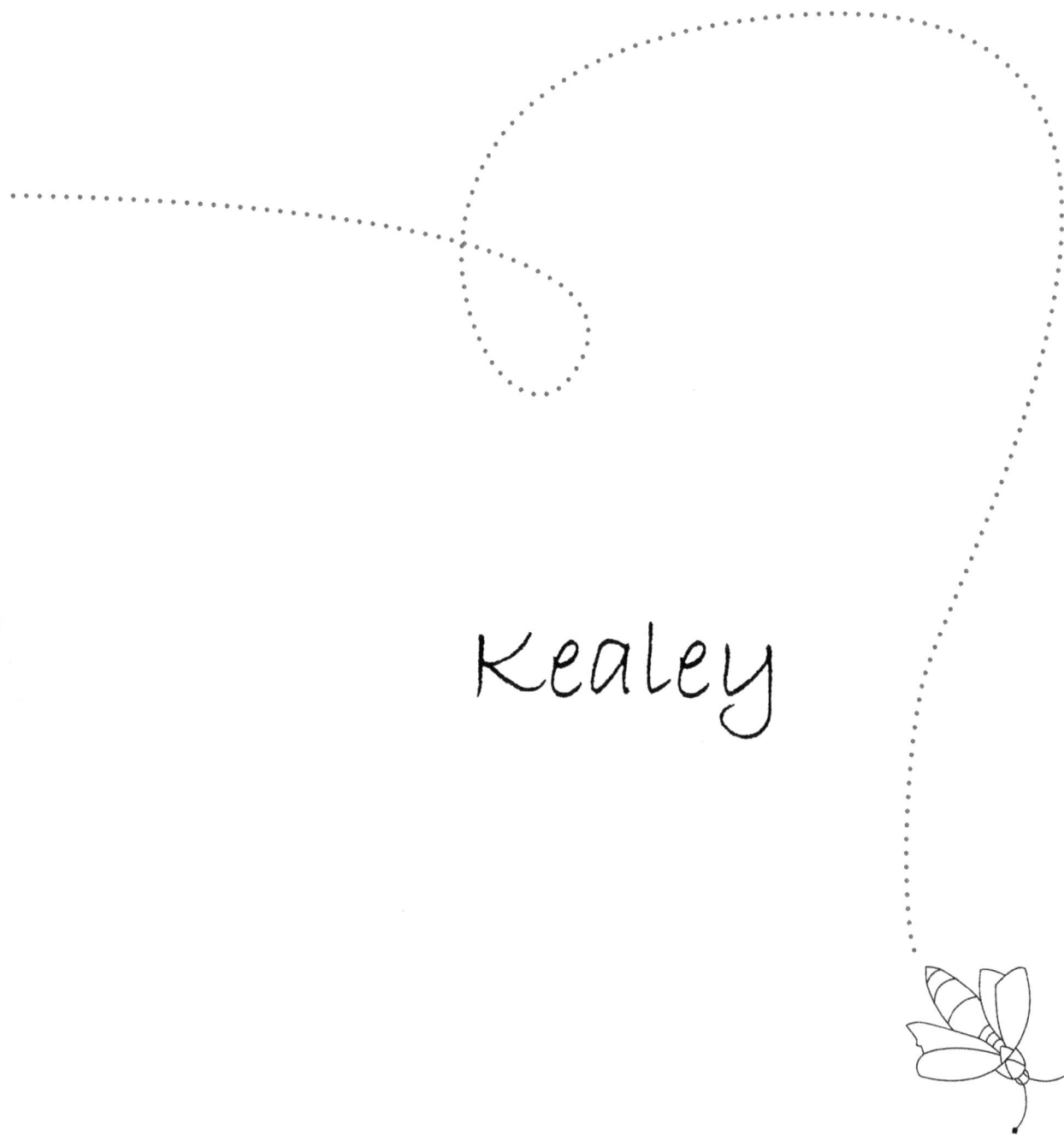

Kealey

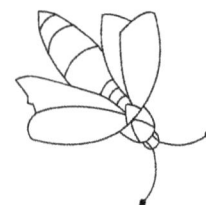

I was born in San Francisco and have lived in the same house all my life. The house has stayed mostly the same, except when we took on a project of "Do It Yourself" landscaping, turning our mediocre backyard into the trampoline "paradise" it is today. That was the summer of 2008.

I love my friends, sketching and photography, singing harmony and piano. My best friend and I sang a Simon and Garfunkel song for graduation. I have been taking piano for ten years and love to play contemporary classical music.

Fate shocked us by sending my mom a stage IV colon cancer diagnosis in November of 2007. She was a nurse practitioner for UCSF, specializing in the care of frail elders. My mom thought it was really important for elders to have the chance to die peacefully at home. She had been working towards a PhD in nursing. I can still remember the light under her door at 3:00 am, while she was studying interview transcripts and working away at her research papers. I always thought it was funny: she would have been Dr. Nurse had she completed her PhD in nursing. It was spring of 2009 when she passed away in the hospital. I was in sixth grade, and my sister was in the second grade.

My pen pal's cancer journey began with a stage I ovarian cancer diagnosis. But the cancer returned. I wondered if it is hard to tell people about it? I remember it always felt funny to tell people that my mom had cancer, because to me she was just my mom.

Hearing about her ovarian cancer brought back memories. I remember how difficult it was to watch my mom go through all the tests. But I also remember the times when we would get good news, and our lives were filled with hope. It must have been so hard to learn that my pen pal was fighting something that she thought she had already defeated.

Before my mom was really sick, I was skeptical of God and also quick to judge the religious. Facing her death completely opened my mind to faith. I am not a "practicing" anything. We celebrate things like Christmas, but I wasn't raised with any religion. Nevertheless, I believe that there is a God. I used to believe that God was a representation of everyone who loved you, but my perspective has changed. I believe first and foremost that God is someone who I pray to.

As I read over my pen pal's letters, I was struck with admiration. We all have troubles, but I have a lot of respect for her courage and quiet (yet resilient) hope in her own hardships. Her kind words and faith encourage me to work harder at resolving conflicts and not worry so much about small things in my school life.

The thing that always struck me as strange, especially after my mom passed away, was how people's lives just always kept going on around me. You could be going in for a huge test that changes your life for better or for worse, but no one would know from the outside. Everyone just keeps going to work, going to school; nothing changes, but everything changes.

As I wrap up this letter, I am thinking about how it is one of the last ones I will write. I just want to say that my pen pal has truly inspired me with her gentle and kind words. So I am thankful for that. I have never even had a real pen pal before. To be perfectly honest, this was wonderful.

~Kealey

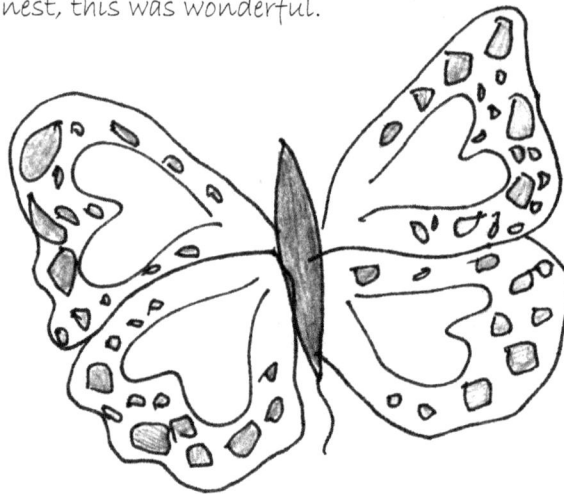

Kealey's mom participated in the Firefly Project and then passed away before she was able to participate in the Adaptation, so Kealey's dad read from her letters for her. What an amazing legacy that Kealey also wanted to participate in Firefly.

Jill & Alicia

My name is Jill. I am 17 years old and live with my mother, sister, and two Cavalier King Charles Spaniels. I lost my dad to cancer two years ago, so I have a bit of an idea of the treatment effects and how hard they are. But on a happier note, I love music, cooking, writing, reading, fashion, films and just having fun.

I was told that you work with sex offenders, which is so interesting because I have been thinking about going into law and becoming a criminal defense attorney.

~ Jill

I am so sorry about the loss of your father. It is such a painful process to watch someone go through treatment and then lose them. And right in the middle of trying to figure out how to be a teenager; that must have been very, very hard. My stepdaughter was 15 when I was diagnosed, and I know that she had a hard time with it, especially since her mom had breast cancer also. It takes a really long time for life to start feeling "normal" again, and then it is not the same normal that it was before.

I have found there have been a lot of gifts that have come out of suffering, but it takes a long time to get that perspective. I was diagnosed with breast cancer six years ago, and treatment was really hard. I am okay at the moment, though I don't take anything for granted anymore. Recognizing how fragile my existence is has made me much more appreciative of how beautiful the world is, and how precious.

Hopefully, by the end of May, I will have completed my doctorate and be a full-fledged psychologist. I work in a clinic where we treat patients who just got out of prison, state or federal, for various kinds of offenses. I treat sexual offenders but also do substance abuse and general mental health treatment.

~ Alicia

I used to be pretty cynical about cancer treatment as clearly there wasn't enough treatment to help my dad, but now I have learned that the treatment was effective for my dad as most pancreatic cancer victims don't survive longer than a year; my dad lived with it for three years. At least your story has a happy ending. I think I am still looking for the gifts that have come out of suffering, and I am trying to be more open to these gifts.

~ Jill

I can't imagine the suffering you and your family went through; the only solace I can imagine is that you had those three years together. I read a blog where one woman talked about how awful it was to go through treatment with no guaranteed outcomes, and another woman responded to her by talking about a friend who died in a car accident. She thought her friend would have chosen cancer as opposed to an accident, as it would have given her a chance to spend more time with the people she loved. That was really important for me to remember. I had time to let everyone I loved know how much I cared, and I still do that. I don't take people or experiences for granted, and that helps me stay more in the moment.

I think it is impressive that you are looking for gifts from the suffering you and your family experienced. You are too young to have to look at such deep questions.

~ Alicia

Recently, I have been thinking about my dad and wondering what advice he would give me about the whole college process. I am so glad that I was introduced to you and was able to participate in this because it has turned around my perspective on cancer. When my dad died I was very negative and pessimistic. How could I not be after watching my dad pass away? But writing to you has helped me redevelop my positive, optimistic attitude. This year has flown by, and I am so happy I have gotten to learn and talk to you in the process, Alicia.

~ Jill

Your dad would be so proud of you, Jill. Knowing that you can be knocked off your feet and that you have the inner strength to get back up, that is undefeatable strength. I am so glad that you regained your optimism.

~ Alicia

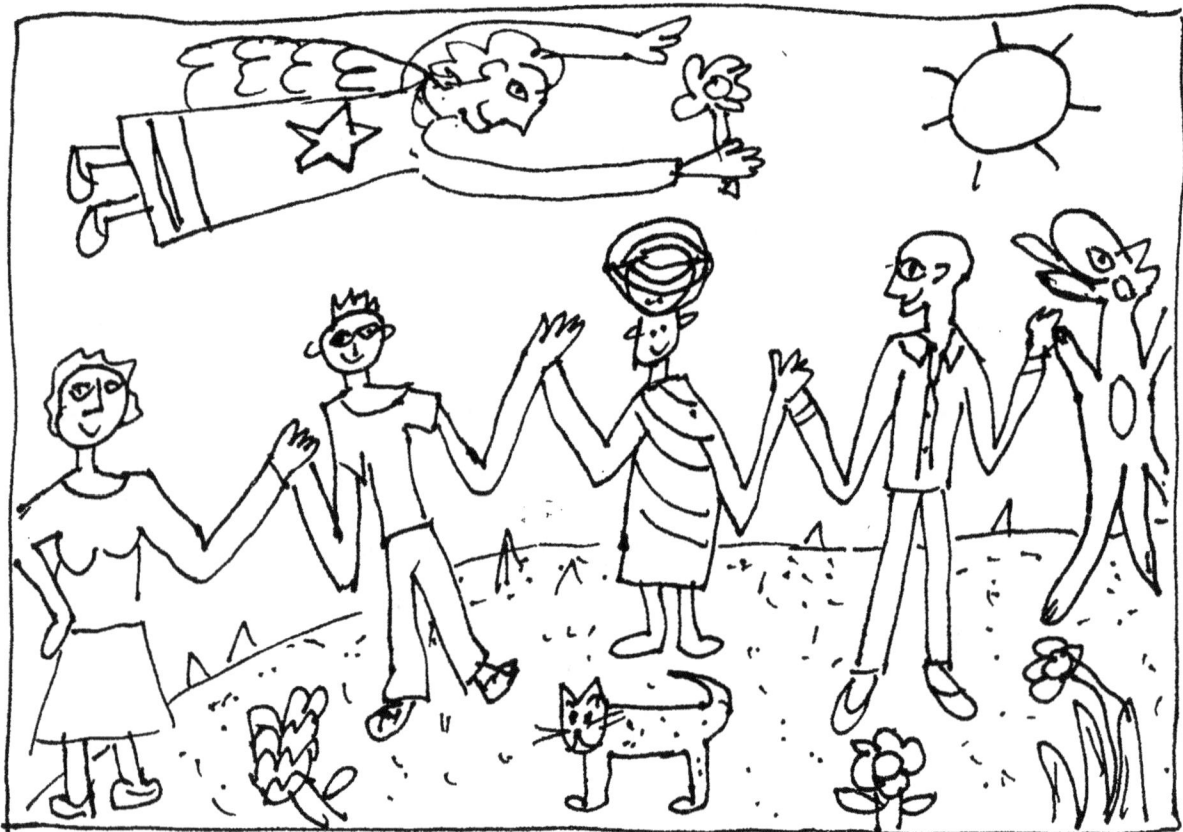

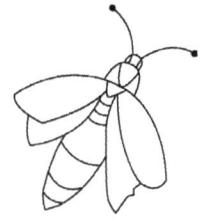

Sophie & Janet

You have no idea how excited I am to write to you, as this is my fifth year in the Firefly Project. Never has anyone's bio ever resounded so much with me as yours did. Both my grandmother and childhood best friend suffered a loss of mobility before they died of cancer, and I remember feeling so incapable of helping them.

A lot of the hurt I feel when I think of my grandmother comes from feeling like I didn't show her how much I loved her often enough when she was healthy. I was too afraid of admitting to her that I knew she was unwell, once she was sick. It hurts me a lot to think that she might have had to doubt the extent of my love for her because I distanced myself, because I didn't know what else to do when she got really sick in the last month of her life. I guess I am really just asking how being physically compromised by cancer affected your mentality, and what kind of support would have been ideal for you?

About me: I am applying to college, I am pretty introspective even though I am loud, and I am strange. I care about almost all music, aesthetics, and surrounding myself with beauty. Salsa is my favorite type of dance, and I am really passionate about pursuing population control by educating women and men to the extent that they will listen.

~ Sophie

When I first read your letter, I actually thought you were a medical or nursing student because you seem so mature. Looking back on my younger days, I wish I had the maturity you seem to have. But that is something that cancer taught me – to be more physically, emotionally and psychologically mature.

I was 34 years old, and single when I was diagnosed, and I had a somewhat conservative surgery because I wanted to keep my fertility. There was a ton of uncertainty about my cancer, and they thought I had uterine and borderline ovarian cancer. After the first surgery they found out it had spread, so I had to have a full hysterectomy in 2010.

I am Christian, and I believe that God got me through cancer. I also believe it happened for a reason and that gave me a lot of peace, although I am still struggling with the infertility part of it.

I have dealt with weight pretty much my whole life. I became obese in college, and so most of my adult life was spent not taking care of my body. Funny, how it took cancer to love my body. After chemotherapy, I was able to lose 110 pounds and currently weigh less than when I was 11 years old. I gained some weight – fine! OWN IT! I am trying to forgive myself.

I think your grandma knew, and still knows, the love you have for her. I just have a feeling.

~ Janet

Right now I am in the midst of the college process, which has sadly forced me to take the outlook where I wonder how whatever I do, or don't do, or think, or say makes me look in the eyes of admission officers, or anyone else around me. This scary thing has started to happen where I think about how I am being evaluated. Then I start to think about the fact that if I am not good enough for the universities, I must just be egregiously underwhelming. It is very twisted and completely untrue, I know, but things like that have a way of filtering into your subconscious.

This all sounds very negative and very self-indulgent, I realize, but the point of sharing this with you is to thank you for talking about body image in your letter. I truly think learning to love all of yourself is a process. I am glad that I have decided to put my energy into making myself valuable to myself rather than try to be validated by others.

~ Sophie

College admissions, like so many things, including illness, are often out of your control. We do our best, and then it is all out of our hands.

~ Janet

I wish there was some way I had the power to support you, Janet, in whatever way you need. I usually just try to heal myself by listening to Bob Marley. It is hard to imagine myself ever feeling abandoned or lost in a family of Jamaican Reggae artists, so I try to put myself there mentally whenever I can.

I have been blessed lately with a lot of positive things: Bi-Rite ice cream, Bollywood dance classes, sufficient time to sleep, good dreams.

~ Sophie

When I heard the words "you have cancer", I learned how important it was to take care of my body. When my mom was dying, I learned how important it was to tell people that I love them as often as I could. Since my mom's passing, my father and I have grown a lot closer for the first time in my life. Most importantly, I love myself more now than ever before cancer. Cancer, illness, death, it all sucks, but it gave me "me."

Here are a few things that I have been happy about, Sophie: *The Big Bang Theory*, my Wednesday lunches with dad, teaching abacus, accepting my ADD and reprogramming my brain not to think of it as a defeat, dark chocolate with sea salt and you. On that cheesy note, I will close my letter!

~ Janet

I have some wonderful news to share! I got into Brown and could not be happier! I had prepped myself for disappointment and was really convinced that I wouldn't get in; I had to read the letter three times before the good news sunk in. I was so overwhelmed that I then took a shower and fell asleep immediately.

~ Sophie

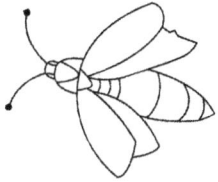

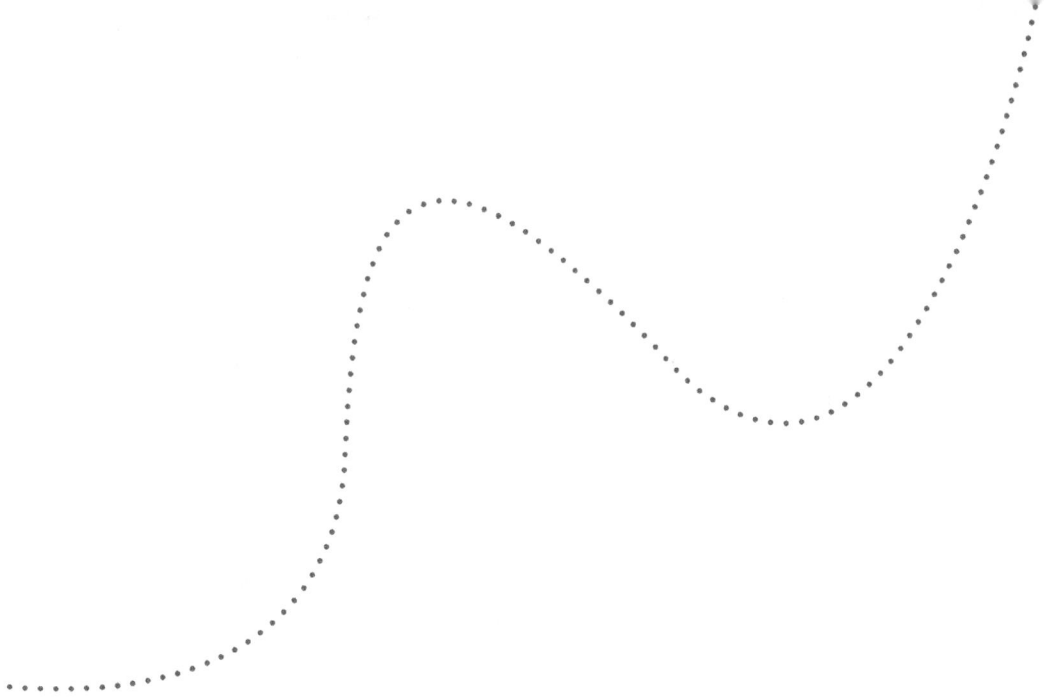

Elena

My pen pal, Michele is now under Hospice Care, and, of course, couldn't be here tonight. Her mom wrote to me because Michele could no longer write. She thought it was amazing that although Michele and I had never met each other face to face, we were so connected.

At the age of 32, my pen pal was diagnosed with stage II breast cancer. Her twins were four years old when she was diagnosed, so they have been living with this all their lives. Currently she is fighting her fourth battle with breast cancer. She prayed that she would get better and knew that she probably would not get her hair back because of the radiation to her brain. This makes her sad because she had beautiful dark brown hair. Being a hairstylist, she loved beautiful hair. She said that her doctor told her if there was anything she wanted to do, to "do it now." She asked what I would want to do. She is praying for a miracle.

When I read her letter I cried so hard, because I am so sorry she has to go through all this. Michele has given me inspiration to be my best. I want her to know that I am rooting for her to beat this and not to be afraid.

Do it now. I asked my stepmother what she would do, and she said she would throw herself a party with everyone she loved and celebrate her life. My dad said he would surround himself with his family and write letters to his future grandchildren, telling them about his life. And my mom said she would do her favorite things – a little each day – like drawing in the morning, and taking walks on the beach, and she would do little acts of kindness each day.

I told Michele in my letter to smile as much as possible and celebrate life. It is really unfair that she is so sick, and I am happy over here. It makes me feel sad and almost guilty.

~ Elena

Imani 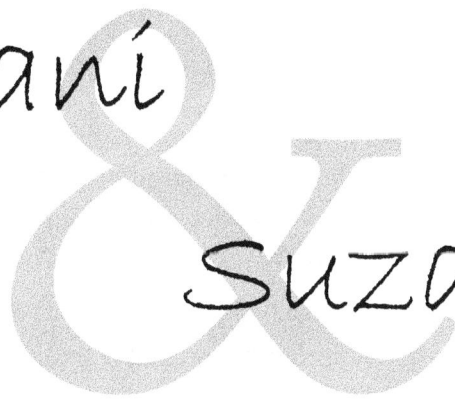 Suzanne

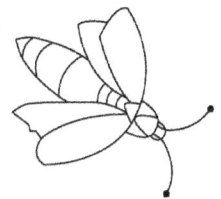

I enjoy helping others in any way I can, whether it is lending a hand as a volunteer or working at camp with children. I am a member of the cheerleading team, Yearbook Club and Burl Toler Scholars and First Graduate, which is a program that helps me be the first in my family to graduate from College.

I am very close with my mother and father, even though they don't live under the same roof. I live with my mother and brother in Hunter's Point, full of cars, pedestrians and sometimes loud music on Friday nights. As a teenager in my household, I do almost everything but cook. I clean the living room, kitchen, my room, the bathrooms, the hallway, and weed whack the back yard. But, I really want to learn how to cook. You are lucky you learned how to cook at a young age.

How are you dealing with your illness, and what is it specifically?

~ Imani

I am 49 years old, and this is significant for me, since my own mother never made it to this age – she died 17 days before her 49th birthday from breast cancer. I was 16 at the time. This is also significant, because I was diagnosed with Breast Cancer too. That is just one part of my life, though. I am married to a good man. He is supportive and funny. I have a 29-year-old daughter, who is much different than I am. She is a girly-girl and likes to get her nails done, shop and buy jewelry. I buy most of my clothes from the thrift store.

I love to cook. I became in charge of the cooking in the house after our mother died. I am in the middle of nine siblings.

How exciting it will be to be the first to graduate from college in your family. Your family must be so proud of you. I was 32 years old when I finished college. Walking up to get my diploma was one of the greatest feelings I have felt.

I would love to hear about you. What is important to you in your life? Where have you traveled?

~ Suzanne

I usually spend the holidays with my dad, but this year, I helped my mom with the cooking. And I didn't know that it was so much work with timing, mixing, heating, preparing, cooling – but it was well worth it.

What do you think it means to have faith, Suzanne?

I have traveled to Paris and Africa, and I personally felt the most at home in Dakar. Getting off the long plane ride from Spain to Senegal, I could taste the heavy hot air, but felt as if I belonged there. At the airport it seemed like we all had signs on our foreheads that said 'Americans': "Sista, brotha, sista – you buy, you buy." But Dakar is so beautiful and full of hard working people; if I could get a chance to go back, I would.

~ Imani

Yes, cooking is a lot of work, with the timing and all, but it is all worth it, like you said. In the Buddhist culture, cooking is said to be one of the highest forms of art because you make it then it goes away by eating it.

I looked up your name because I was intrigued with it. It means faith, belief. The meaning makes it even more wonderful. Please tell your mom or dad or whomever named you that it is a beautiful name, Imani.

I did not quite understand what it meant to have faith as a young girl. Then my mother died, and my faith as I knew it slid away. Now as an adult, I have faith in life and myself. Since my second diagnosis, my faith is even stronger.

~ Suzanne

Chapter 3

This Is Not What I Had Planned

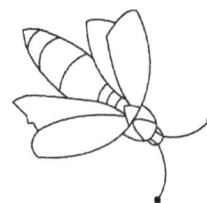

Molly & Tatjana

I love many things, especially water. I think water is one of the most pleasing things to my senses in all respects: touch, sound, sight and taste. I suppose smell too. I especially love freezing cold water; it makes me feel so alive and real. I value honesty and genuine connections. I heard you like to dance. I love to dance too, and I do theater, but it is not something I am especially interested in. I don't really fear very many things in the arena of risk taking. This summer I went on a five-week trip to Laos and Cambodia, on which I could only bring five items in addition to essential toiletries. I am eager to experience as much as I can.

~ Molly

I am a big fan of honesty and genuine connections. I have lived all my life that way, but I am trying to get even better at it. I want to learn from all the pain I went through with my ex-husband, and be more truthful to myself, and stand up more for myself and what I need to have in my life to be happy. Uh, that sounded like a very serious beginning of this very first letter.

Dancing makes me happy and feel alive, Molly. I already liked dancing when I was your age and coming from a poor family, I was able to get a stipend to go to dance school. Moving the body to the rhythm of music and turning off all thoughts makes me incredibly happy; it always has. Why did you decide to participate in Firefly?

~ Tatjana

I am sorry to hear about the divorce you are going through. That sounds like such an acute type of pain – to think you have found the most powerful love connection of your life and to later realize it wasn't so.

College applications are a big part of my life at the moment. I can feel a sense of general depression among the other seniors. Writing the essays with the idea that I have to change the way I present myself is so against my ethic.

It's hard for me to accept the idea that I have to decide which qualities about myself are most attractive to these people that I don't particularly care about; the qualities like kindness or capacity to love have nothing to do with these college applications, and finally that all of these things determine where I will spend the next four years of my life.

What makes me happy? I had to learn to make myself happy. I wrote a lot in my journal, listened to music. I also learned to find beauty in the condition of feeling things, including sadness. When I spent time alone in the city, I learned how to spend time alone, thinking, noticing and pursuing whims, talking to whomever I met.

I participated in the Firefly Project two years ago and had a positive experience. My mom is also a breast cancer survivor, and a lot of my family members have died from cancer, too.

~ Molly

I am officially a single woman with my own last name again as of December 31st, 2011. What an auspicious date! To start the New Year as a new person, it is bittersweet, Molly. I emailed my co-workers informing them of my new (old) name and one asked, "Is it something to celebrate?" and I, not thinking, said "Yes." But then she said something very thoughtful instead of congratulating me: "I am sorry your marriage didn't work out." And I think that pretty much reflects the feelings that I am having.

I am totally open to talk about anything regarding my cancer. I have to say that I don't really remember too much from the period. All the chemotherapy and drugs make me remember only a lot of fog. Brain fog makes concentrating difficult and memories shady. What was much worse than the chemo was the estrangement from my husband at the same time. I felt as if I was running against a wall and not getting to the other side. I felt abandoned and betrayed. How could he leave me when I was feeling so bad, and I needed him? That was me then. Now, I am much, much better. But I still don't understand.

~ Tatjana

I am both sorry and glad to hear about your marriage officially ending. I imagine it must be a time of mixed emotions. It must have been difficult to feel yourself losing your mental faculties during your cancer treatment. Sometimes during emotional stress, I feel like I am losing my acuity, and it scares me quite a bit.

For the first time in my adolescence, I am not sure what the most important goal is for me right now. Overall, my goal is to be happy, to surround myself with special, wonderful, loving people in a strong community and always maintain verve for life. But right now I am living in a very different way than I usually do, with little thought or planning. Just seeing what happens. Tatjana, it has been great writing to you.

~ Molly

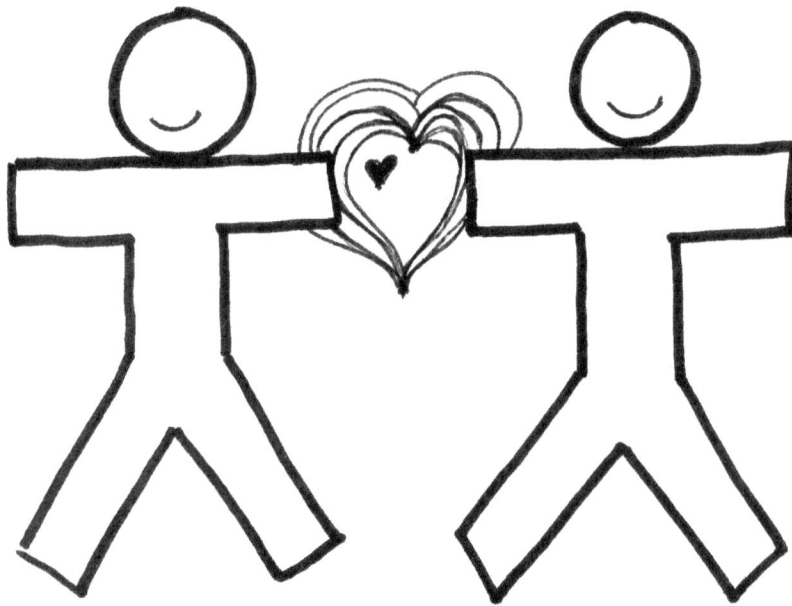

Andrea & Barbara

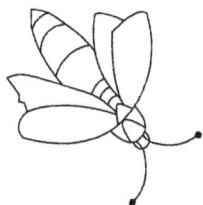

I have lived in San Francisco my whole life. Where are you from? Next year I am going to be an Aggie at UC Davis and will be playing on the golf team. I have a twin sister, and both my parents are from China. They both moved here as kids, and all my grandparents live in the City. My grandparents actually cook dinner for us on weekdays, so I get to have amazing Chinese food every night.

I was told you had uterine cancer. What happens when you have uterine cancer? Do they have to remove your uterus? My dad had lymphoma three times, but he doesn't really like to talk about the times he had cancer or what he went through which is hard for me because I am interested about what it was like.

~ Andrea

I am doing very well, Andrea. My last chemo was nearly a year ago and everything is good so far. I am sorry to hear that your father had to go through this. I am only guessing, but I think your father is being protective of you and your sister in not wanting to discuss it. It is something my dad would have done in a similar situation.

~ Barbara

My twin sister and I will be parting ways. I will be going off to UC Davis, and my sister will be across the country at Princeton to play golf. It is definitely going to be a change because we have never been so far away from each other for such a long time. However, it will be good for us to gain our independence – and what better time than college? I will only be two hours away from the City, far enough to get away from my parents, but close enough so I can still come home for home-cooked meals and laundry.

~ Andrea

I understand about being far away from your sister. I was diagnosed in 2010 with endometrial cancer. My primary care physician suggested I go to the University of Colorado in Denver since I wanted to be near my sister. I was given chemotherapy and started to lose my hair about two weeks after the first treatment. Within the next few weeks, I had lost my eyebrows and eye lashes too. I have had a few side effects. I have neuropathy in my feet, and I no longer wear high heels. I have chemo-brain, and I can no longer do the job I have had for over 30 years. This is not what I had planned.

~ Barbara

I have never heard of chemo-brain before – is this common? Do you have trouble remembering things or can you not remember things from the past? I talked to my dad a little about his cancer. I used to wonder if he was in pain. I know he went vegan for a while after the treatment to cleanse his system, and I remember very specifically that my grandma would make him special vegan pot stickers.

The third time he got it, he would go to the hospital every Friday for about five hours and get his treatment. Then he would pick us up from school, always with a big smile, and take us for a snack, and then he would take us golfing. It was never about him, but about us, and I am so happy he is cancer-free now.

~ Andrea

I am beginning this letter in the waiting room at UCSF for my three-month follow up appointment. Happily I got good news, Andrea. No change. No evidence of disease. It is always a relief to hear those words. Chemo-brain affects my thinking process, especially when under stress. I still cannot read a book and remember what I have read. It is difficult for me to learn new things. Not all patients get chemo-brain. I don't know why, but something triggered in my brain. It was very frightening for me at first as I didn't understand why I no longer knew how to do things which had been almost second nature.

~ Barbara

Life is about our daily triumphs over hardships, and you seem to be doing just that. I am truly amazed about the strength that you and other cancer patients have.

~ Andrea

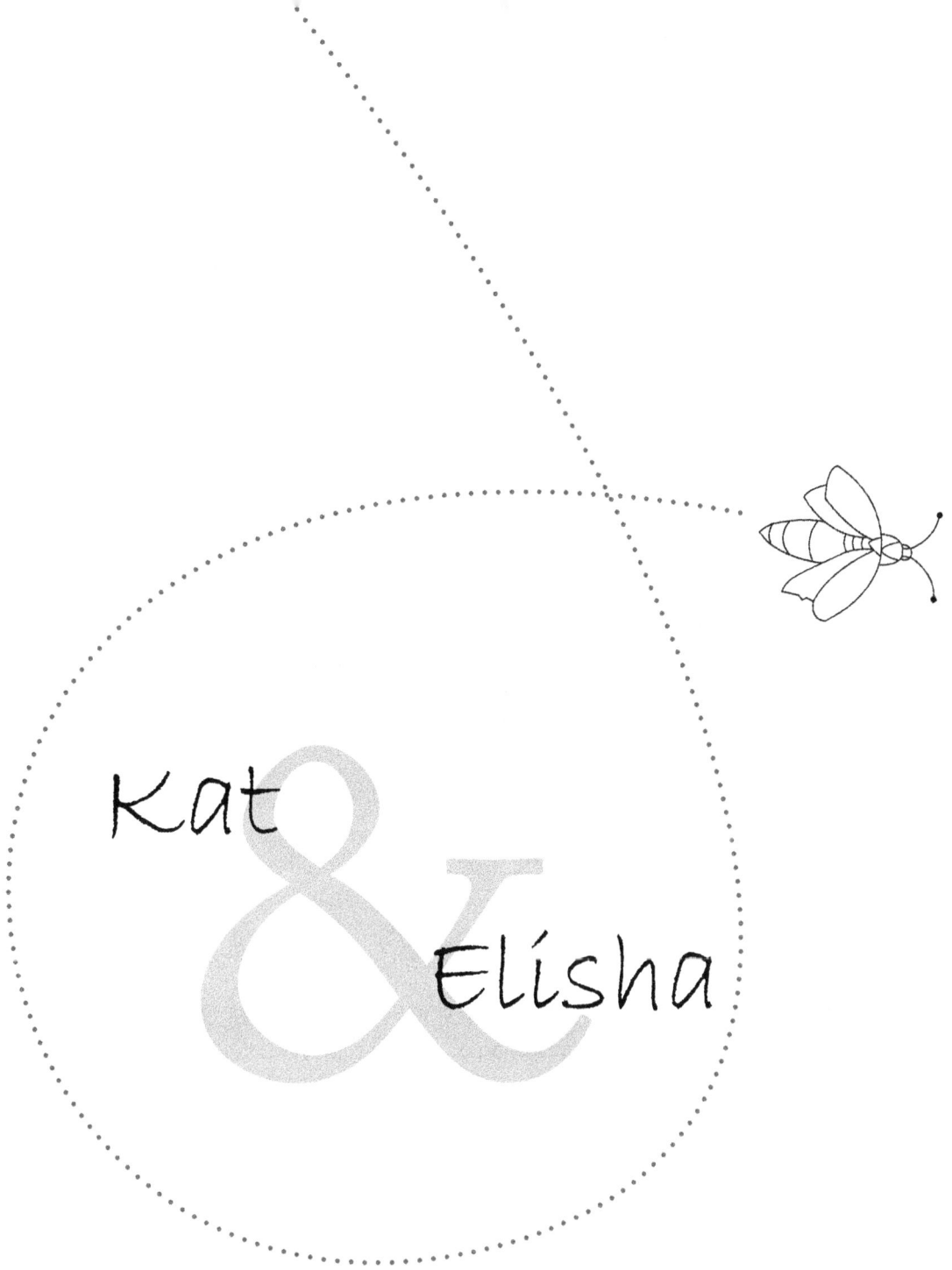

Kat & Elisha

At the moment I am taking four AP classes, I am captain of my water polo team, president of the Cancer Awareness Club, and choosing between two colleges, both of which are recruiting me. I am learning towards Bucknell, but my parents are strongly encouraging Brown.

My dad films, watches and supports every water polo game I play, and he has made athletics so much fun for me throughout my life. He rowed crew in the 1984 Los Angeles Olympics, and I have always held myself to his to the standard, which I might someday reach.

What are your feelings and point of view on life now that it has been put to the test? I am not really sure how to start this conversation, as I don't know where we will end up, or what we will find is important to talk about.

~ Kat

I remember my senior year of high school, and I can't say I miss being that stressed about school and life decisions.

I had a biopsy over the winter break during my freshman year of college, and that was when they found the cancer cells in my breast. After my surgery the only treatment I had was Zoladex, an ovarian suppression drug. It basically made me go through a temporary menopause, but nothing debilitating. I began school again that July at Berkeley, and life pretty much went back to normal.

I love overcast days in the fall; I just love the feeling. I am not sure why because most people don't like those gloomy days.

~ Elisha

So, I made a college choice: Bucknell! I am so excited about it, and I think my parents are finally warming up to the idea. It was probably the hardest decision I have ever had to make in my life!

The switch from UCLA to Berkeley must have been hard, especially after surgery. Were you ever scared? Recently there was another suicide at my school, making it the third one in my four years. Does having been sick with a disease that could potentially kill you make you mad that people take their own lives when every day others are having their lives taken from them by illnesses, wars, violence, etc.? I felt really angry and sad when I first found out about the suicide. I could just not understand why someone would do that.

~ Kat

I think I was more scared starting at UCLA than I was switching to Berkeley, or even going through surgery.

I know getting my wisdom teeth removed was ten times scarier than getting a mastectomy! For some reason the dental work was far more nerve racking than the breast cancer surgery.

It is always so sad to hear about someone taking his or her life. I don't think my experience makes me mad at people who take their own life. I just wish there was something that someone could have done to help them.

~ Elisha

I was just thinking that second semester senior year is so overrated!

~ Kat

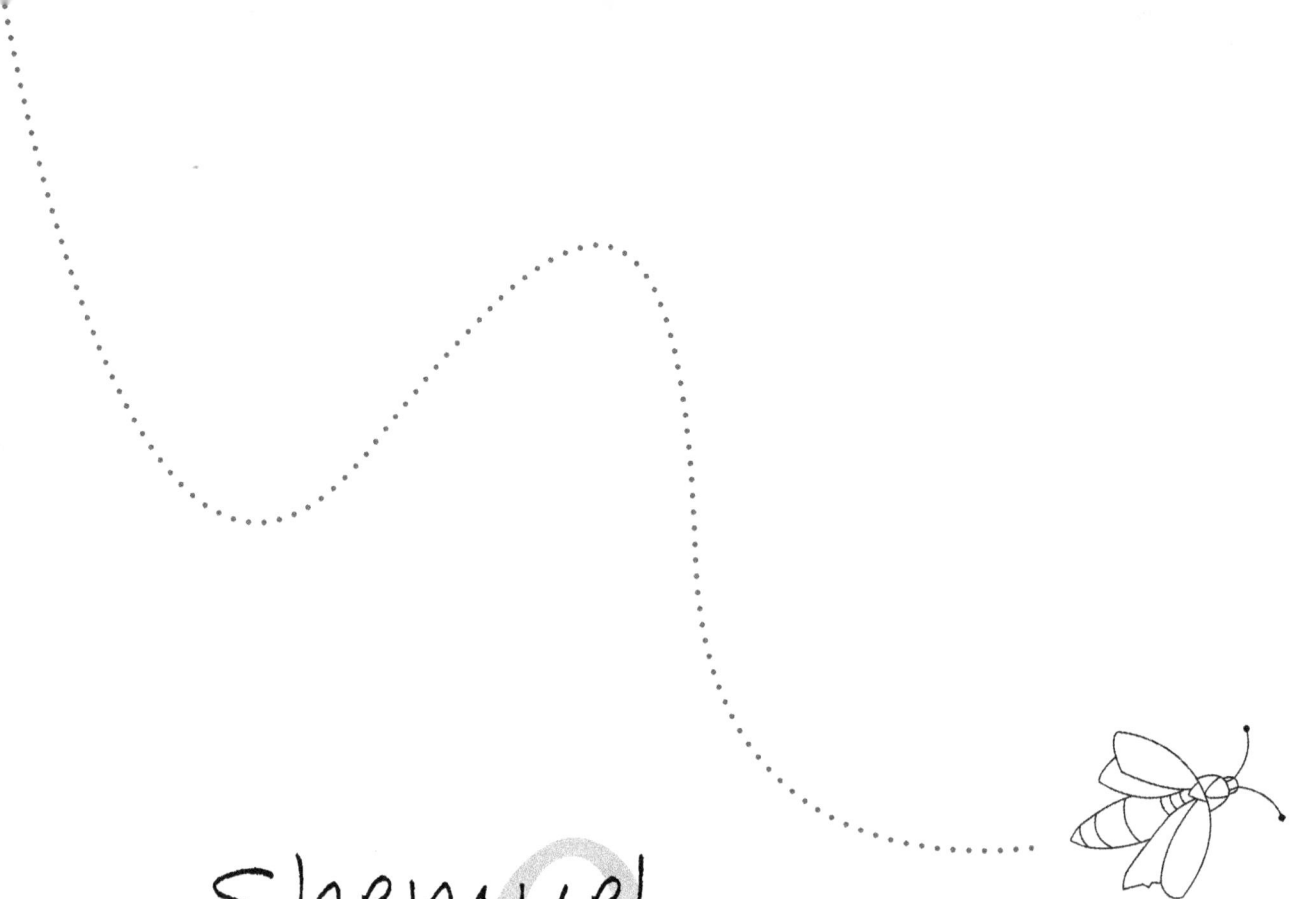

Shemuel

&

Todd C.

My family and I are originally from Singapore, and we moved to Indiana in 1999, but came to San Francisco when I was seven years old.

What kind of cancer do you have? How is it to have cancer? To be honest when people hear that someone has cancer, all they know is that it is extremely hard to cure, but some people, including me, don't know all the symptoms – or the feelings that go along with it.

~ Shemuel

In 2008, I was diagnosed with acute lymphoblastic leukemia and lymphoma. Similar to any adversary, the more you know the better prepared you are to defeat it. During this period, I devoted all my time and focus on improving health and saving my life, and I continue to do so. This meant multiple extended stays in the hospital (14 to 28 days or more.) Regular life seems distant during this period due to the susceptibility to viruses, infections and other health risks that most people handle without thinking. In short, Cancer has shown its face in my life, and I will be on my best behavior and ready if it wants to tangle with me again!

While in treatment, I did what I could to remain interested and engaged in exercise and movement in whatever forms safe and appropriate. The exercise bike in my hospital room was essential to achieving this.

~ Todd C.

It was very informational to know what exactly happens when people have cancer. I only knew that the patient spends a long time in the hospital and goes through Chemotherapy. Todd, as a teenager, I associate cancer as a life threatening disease, but I do not have much more in-depth knowledge than that.

I feel that preventing cancer in any way possible should be exercised for our future. My mom read about how using the microwave can give you cancer. At first this sounded like a joke, but I respect that my mom is concerned about my health, so now I only use the microwave to make popcorn.

As I mentioned, I am from Singapore. At the age of 18, it is mandatory for all Singaporean male citizens to undergo two years in the army. I feel like that will give me the physical exercise to stay fit and keep healthy.

~ Shemuel

The truth is, cancer is part of a healthy unaffected person as much as it is part of a person with disease. Our bodies have tools to manage free-radicals and help us to follow a normal cell life cycle.

I consider myself like a garden and consider how I want to grow until the crop fruit dies and is replanted again.

~ Todd C.

A few of my parent's friends have been diagnosed with cancer over the past few years so I have been more in contact with it. We have also been studying cancer in biology class, explaining how tumors are a result of cancer and so forth.

~ Shemuel

Cancer seems to be playing a larger part in people's lives these days. When I was young, I thought older people just died of *old age*. As if *old age* was something to be afraid of when there are so many other things that can kill us.

~ Todd C.

When people say that they have cancer, most people do not quite know how to react besides knowing that it is an incurable disease. After talking with you and other people with cancer, I feel that I should explore the world more and experience as much as I can. I am learning so much from you!

~ Shemuel

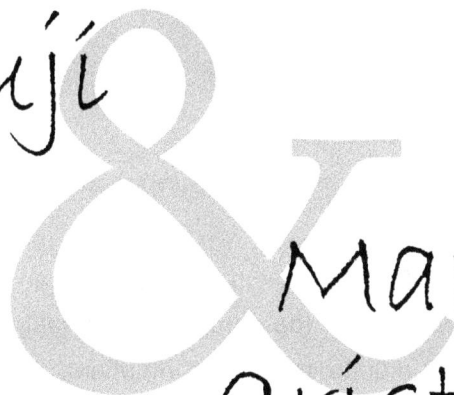

Puji & Maria Cristina

I have one younger sister, whom I love dearly despite our endless arguments. I have been playing soccer for 11 years and have been learning and performing Indian classical dance for ten years. I got my driver's license almost six months ago and am still rejoicing in my liberty. I tutor younger students, and I strive to maintain a positive attitude about all aspects of my life.

I know you may be wondering why I have chosen not to say anything in regards to your sickness. Some people deal with their obstacles by talking about them constantly, while for some it brings them strength to pretend their problems don't exist. While I don't know how you are dealing with your condition, I am here to listen, advise, or distract you, basically benefit you in any and every way possible. Either way you are in my prayers, and I wish you all the best in the war with your illness.

What are your goals and dreams? What scares you?

~ Puji

Does your name mean anything, Puji? From your letter, I can say that we are already friends. One of my goals is to learn the computer. It is taking me too long to learn. Sitting in a chair and facing a monitor makes me impatient.

I feel challenged. Chemotherapy left an effect on me for sure. I can't see very well, and I used to have 20/20 vision. My sense of smell is limited as well as my sense of taste. But I still give life my all. I am just grateful I am not all wiped out.

What scares me...I am really afraid that I will fail as a mom. I don't expect my children to be perfect, but I hope I have given them the tools to lead a good life. I am also afraid of hurting people's feelings. My goal in my heart is to press on to do the right thing above the standards of this world and to be kind.

What are you afraid of?

~ Maria Cristina

My full name, Pujitha, means goddess in Sanskrit, but no one calls me Pujitha, except for my mom and dad when they are mad.

I am sure it must be very fulfilling to take pride in the success of your kids. I know my mother worries about how she is bringing me up. She feels nervous and guilty for any possibility of failure in my life. I am fascinated by the immense amount of possibility within a computer. I have helped my parents adapt to the new technology too. Good for you for starting to learn.

I am a person who can't stand to sit still. I need to constantly be doing something. As a high school student, I find there is so much pressure to be successful, to get good grades, to be popular, to get into a good college. So I guess you could say, I am afraid of failing, or worse, letting my parents down even though they constantly tell me that there is nothing I could do to make them ever stop loving me.

~ Puji

I can tell your parents must be so proud of you. I feel, Puji, that overall I have been given a gift. My friends, my home, my kids, even my enemies are my gifts. I am fortunate that I have gotten through these last years. I didn't have money to buy Christmas gifts for my kids this year, but I am lucky that they understand. I thank God for everything. I very much appreciate your friendship, too.

~ Maria Cristina

I have asked my mother to keep you in her prayers. Your gratefulness inspired me and makes me feel petty for my high school stress and difficulties, but I imagine I should be grateful for having such simple problems.

~ Puji

Your parents did a great job raising you! I will miss receiving the big white envelope with your letter amongst the smaller intimidating envelopes with bills in them. May God in heaven continuously bless you and your family,

~ Maria Cristina

Chapter 4
This Time Around

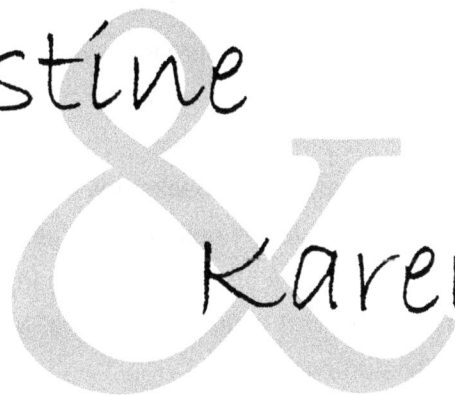

Christine
&
Karen K.

I can describe myself as happy no matter what circumstances I am in. I always try to make others smile, and I can also be very quiet and shy at times.

I decided to join Firefly because I thought it would be a great way of meeting someone who has been through a lot and can find a way to share their story. I want to get to know you bit by bit. How do you feel about this? How are you feeling at this point, reading my letter?

~ Christine

You are now part of my journey. We are on it together.

I am an artist. These days I have been working with clay, and I have taught ceramics for many years. I am a painter as well and how I approach my glazes reflects that. Those are two things that I can remember doing and enjoying as far back as nursery school.

Let me start by giving you a little of my cancer backstory. In 2003, I was diagnosed with leukemia. Leukemia is a blood cancer. It was quite a shock. At that moment I knew that my life had turned a corner. Nothing would be the same from there on in. That was when the journey began. I cried. I laid in bed listening to music. Music has sustained me. It inspires, it consoles. It is transforming.

I received a bone marrow transplant on November 19th, 2005, two years from the date of my diagnosis. My donor was anonymous. That date is now considered my new second birthday. I will be 60 years old soon. I hope one day to meet my donor and thank her. We are sisters. Without her stem cells, I do not think I would be alive today.

I am not out of the woods yet. A bone marrow transplant can kill you. There is a long period of adjustment as the new immune system gets to know the new body, learning to coexist to live with each other in peace and harmony. It is a balancing act. A fine-tuning. I think of it as putting a new transmission in an old car body. I am still in treatment. I will be dealing with this for the rest of my life. And may I live a long life.

~ Karen K.

How does a person get leukemia? Is it inherited or does something happen to a person's body causing them to get it? Do you ever wonder if your life would have been different had you not gotten sick?

~ Christine

My leukemia morphed into a more serious blood disease that would lead to complete marrow failure. That put me on the road to a bone marrow transplant. The donor has to be a close genetic DNA match and can be anywhere in the world. All I know of my donor is that she was 25 years old. There had been a death in her family just before my BMT. Her information is kept confidential for a year. I waited for the cells to do their thing; they seemed to know where to go and what to do. Magic. Every morning the nurses began my day by peeling off a page from the room calendar. And I would ask myself how I was going to get through another day. I was in the hospital a few days shy of a month, Christine.

I now have a new DNA. I have a new sister in the world whose DNA I share. She has saved my life. I know not where or who she is. I am grateful to this generous person. I would one day like to meet and thank her.

My parents are not alive, but I have two sisters. It is a different world with our parents gone. I am kind of glad they are not around for this part of my life. I would worry about them worrying about me. I am glad they didn't have to go through this with me.

~ Karen K.

I am glad that you let me into your life; it is a huge step for someone to open up to a person whom they haven't met. Thank you for actually taking your time and explaining to me how a transplant works.

I hope that you are getting better health-wise and life-wise. I think you are a brave woman for pushing yourself and being determined to fight this. Never give up, Karen. Giving up is not an option!

~ Christine

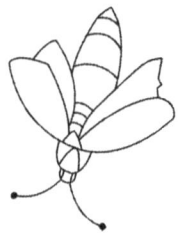

Rachel & Karen K.

I am so happy I have the opportunity to write to you. I am a member of the Cancer Awareness Club at my school. My grandfather passed away from liver cancer, and my dad was diagnosed with colon cancer. He recently had surgery, and we received news that he is cancer free.

I am a member of the swim team, I take and teach dance lessons, I am a senior mentor to freshmen, and I plan retreats at my school and help out with prayer services.

~ Rachel

Wow, it sounds like you have been touched by cancer quite a bit yourself. But, you lead a very active and busy life. You are very engaged in LIFE!

I love clay. What I love the most about it is the transformations it goes through. There is an element of not being in total control when it is in the kiln and firing. That is where the magic happens. The unknowing. And the surprise. It is a metaphor for my life. In November it has been six years since my bone marrow transplant. That is considered a second birthday. Transformation. I am still a work in progress.

When I was in the hospital in the very first days, I received a phone call from an Irish singer I had met years before. She was living in NYC and coming to town to perform and needed a babysitter. That call made me realize that only part of me was in the hospital, and my life had not stopped.

~ Karen K.

I think my dad felt the same way you did. He didn't really want anyone knowing about his cancer for a while. Maybe he didn't want people to pity him or didn't want to admit it to himself. I also kind of felt the same way about his cancer actually. I didn't tell my friends until it came time for the surgery, because I guess I couldn't say it out loud myself.

I think it is cool to have a pen pal. Most days, people don't really talk about themselves, and letter writing is a way that we can share things we don't share every day.

~ Rachel

It feels good to be among the living. I am so appreciative to have lived this long and feel this well. Last year was the year of realizing that I actually am able to look forward; there is a future.

Last year was about taking care of business. Drained to no end. I was dealing with survivor's depression to boot. Health wise I am not out of the woods yet.

The question that it always comes down to is: HOW DO I WANT TO LIVE THE REST OF MY LIFE? What does it mean to have survived this long? Where do I fit in? My priorities have changed. I am my main priority. Taking care of me. And that is not being selfish. I deserve to live. I have changed, but basically I am the same person. I have very few regrets. I will not take any regrets to my grave.

I am still figuring it out. I am completely original. No one has walked on my road in my shoes. I will give myself a lifetime to figure it out.

~ Karen K.

I am getting a little scared to graduate from high school in three months. It is crazy to think I am already leaving. It feels as if I have just gotten here. I still have no clue as to where I am going to school, but hopefully I will know soon.

~ Rachel

I remember my last days of high school. I had been accepted to a college in New Hampshire. I was going on an adventure. It was small. It was wild. I made a lot of art. It was cold, for sure. I was in it for the view and got a vision instead.

You have so many surprises in front of you, Rachel. Be open. Be curious. Be kind. Don't take life too seriously. Most of life is absurd. It is amazing. Life is magic, the way it all fits together. It amazes me.

~ Karen K.

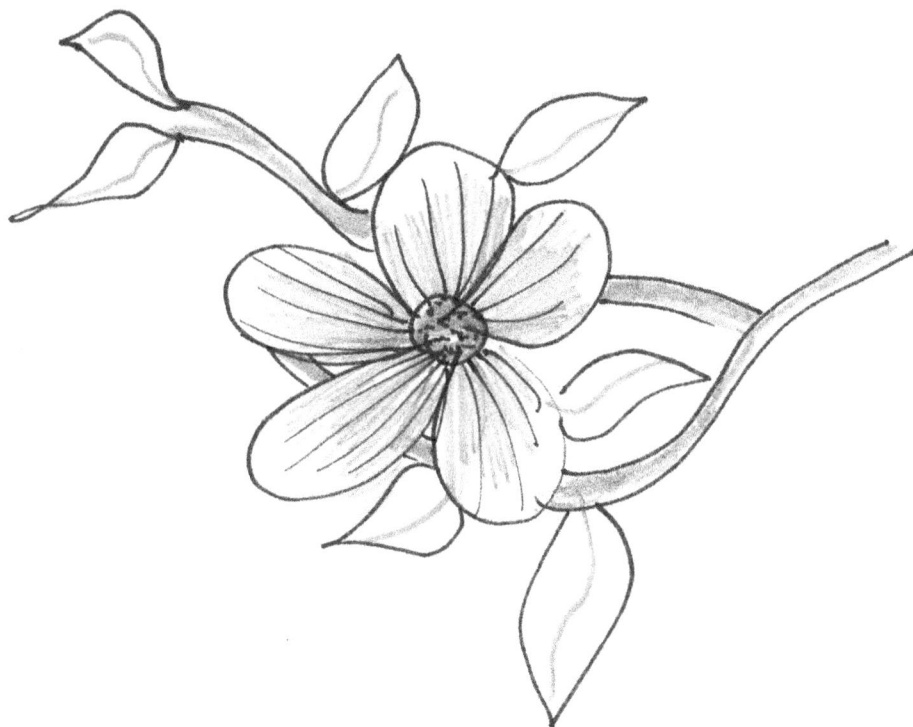

I want to thank you for being my pen pal. This Art for Recovery Firefly Project is a way to talk to someone whom you have never met, yet I feel I can share anything with you. It is a different form of recovery, but a good and healthy way.

~ Rachel

Rebecca

My pen pal is not here tonight, but in the beginning, I told her I would like to write to her about songs that mean something to me. Each song brings up a memory, or a thought, or an image, and I think these snapshots of my past and present define me better than any list of activities or attempts to describe myself. Here are a few:

"The Weight" by The Band: This song reminds me of my father. One year it was the only CD we had in the car for the entire winter and since we go to Tahoe every few weekends, it got played a lot. He'd blast it and sing out of key. If we can sit with each other at five am in the morning, listening to old music and laughing at each other in our tired delirium as we drive through California, I know I have it good.

"Sir Duke" by Stevie Wonder: I played this song in my steel drum band in middle school. Middle school for me was heaven.

"Bleeker Street" by Simon and Garfunkel: When I was younger, my family used to go swimming each weekend in the summer. My dad taught us how to dive over noodles. Then we would go to dinner and get dessert at this frozen yogurt place that looked like a castle. And on the way home, I would fall asleep with my hair still wet listening to this CD that my dad played in the car.

I am a senior in high school, Editor of the newspaper and yearbook. I am a black belt in taekwondo. I love skiing. I have been playing piano forever, but I never practice. I just love it. I love photography, but I can't draw or paint or anything else.

I was interested to hear about my pen pal's cancer journey. My mom went through treatment when I was in the fifth grade and then another surgery for a false alarm. But we didn't talk about it much.

My pen pal and I were meant to be in each other's lives.

~ Rebecca

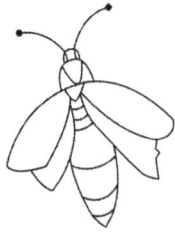

sharon & Kiera

I joined Firefly because I wanted to try to understand my relationship with my younger daughter. After my cancer, my daughter and I had a very challenging relationship, so I thought I might better understand her by communicating with others in her age group. It was such a fulfilling experience last year that I decided to write again this year.

~ Sharon

I bet it is hard for your daughter to cope with the fact that you had to go through treatment and how stressed you were and how stressed she felt also.

I have had to put all my focus on school with finals coming up, basketball, and my parents putting a lot of pressure to start applying for college scholarships in swimming. I just have not had a day to myself.

~ Kiera

Getting older is challenging. I try to act and think "young," but there are times when it just doesn't quite make it, no matter how hard I try. Be positive. I am grateful to wake up every morning and see the sunrise again, of having the opportunity to spend another day on this earth and be with my family and friends.

~ Sharon

Sometimes I feel my life passing by without fun anymore, as if I am becoming an adult before I am finished with being a teenager. My New Year's resolution is to be able to be a calmer person and try not to be so bossy.

~ Kiera

I feel saddened by your letter. When I was going through chemotherapy, I felt completely incapable of being in control of my own life and body and at the mercy of those "deadly" drugs that were being pumped into my body every other week. I could just feel my body getting weaker and weaker and having less and less control. AND there was absolutely nothing I could do about it. YOU do have control over your life.

~ Sharon

Talia & Evalyn

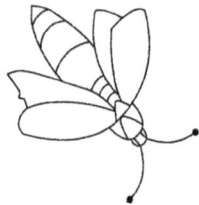

Throughout my life I have never known someone who had cancer. I was extremely enthused when I heard about the Firefly Project because I realized that while everyone has his or her own set of issues and hindrances throughout their lives, cancer is not only extremely difficult to deal with, but is an illness that takes great fortitude to survive every day. I am really interested in the psychological parts of experiences, and constantly attempt to understand others' perspective in life. I truly admire you for sharing such a personal experience.

Although I haven't experienced having cancer, last year I fell while skiing and had surgery on my knee. It ended up being more than just a fall; I had a tibial medial plateau fracture, which basically entailed having two screws in my knee to "fix" the mess. Although it wasn't life threatening, after the surgery I was subjected to being in a wheel chair for about two months. This was especially difficult because I was on the cross-country team, and I love musical theater, and I wasn't able to dance or run track.

Though I am so grateful for the privileged life I have been given, and am blessed for my health, my own misfortunes have shaped me as well.

Throughout high school, I have always felt on the outs. I have friends, participate in many after school activities, and am constantly working hard to strive in school. However, I have had to make an effort to find people who I can really talk to and trust.

~ Talia

I don't even know where to begin to reply to all the amazing and interesting things you told me in your letter. When I got the diagnosis that my seemingly innocuous uterine fibroid had a touch of cancer in it, I filled with fear and panic so quickly I could hardly breathe. Panic stayed with me the entire 100 days I had to deal with it. My 100 days in the caves of cancer. I lost 39 pounds. This was mainly my own artist's mind dramatizing and creating the idea that I was far more ill than I actually was. But that is what people do sometimes; we all fear death so much.

My momma gave me my first blank journal when I was 15 years old, and I have kept personal journals ever since. Interestingly, when I was diagnosed with cancer last summer, I could not write at first because I was too scared. When I got the "all clear," the writing began to pour out of me again.

No matter how difficult it is to do so at times, trust that with courage and perseverance, your creativity and passion will see you through. And you will have more compassion and ability to help others on the other side of the darkness. But you seem to have already learned that valuable and loving truth.

I have been in major Broadway shows, and even received a Tony nomination for one of them some years ago. I adore musical theater still, even though when we moved to San Francisco from New York City 11 months ago, I decided to let myself live the life of a professional writer. I don't miss performing at all!

~ Evalyn

Death is a scary issue that always seems faraway and in the deepest, darkest corners of life. I have recently been thinking a lot about death. A 15-year-old girl who attended another high school committed suicide. I didn't know the girl, but it made me really appreciate all of my close friends, and to want to be there for them.

I can't imagine, Evalyn, how interesting it must be to look back on your "cancer journal" to remind yourself what you went through. I love keeping journals and wrote every night my sophomore year. Although writing in a journal has been painful for me, it is the best way to understand the feelings that I am experiencing and be able to grow from them.

I am so excited to hear about all your Broadway experiences. Do you miss New York? I can't believe you were in "Les Miserables". It is one of my favorite musicals, and I am constantly listening to the music in my car.

~ Talia

I have had many people, dear friends, who have died, of AIDS mostly, cancer a little, other things, and as much as I miss them and was sad at their parting, I have never been so aware of death as I became when I received my cancer diagnosis. I contemplate death a lot in meditation, which according to the Buddha, is one of the main things we should think about since it happens to us all.

My daddy died very, very suddenly with no warning whatsoever when I was in high school. Suddenly our family was a fragile card table with one leg missing, about to topple over any moment. I didn't get over his loss for a very long time. And, I think it made me very frightened of death.

It truly does scare me. I am not so evolved yet that it doesn't hold some terrors for me, even when I go get my three-month check-ups. My cancer was minor, compared to others', but it caused me terrible fear and deep sickening suffering nonetheless, Talia. I am just scared of what I will feel like when the illness gets more serious, no matter what that illness may be. Cancer is a son of a bitch of a disease, but there are so many other ways the human body can succumb, and I am now aware of just how fragile we all are.

What if you choose some songs from Broadway shows you love? Songs that speak to you, say the things you want to say about yourself and your life. Then, when we finally meet, we will get together and sing them!

Pick some songs. I will too. I think my first choice may be "People", from *Funny Girl*. Maybe you and I can even sing a duet?

~ Evalyn

I am someone who loves to be around people and have deep relationships with everyone who is close to me in my life. Although I definitely need alone time, I am totally enthralled by others and am always reaching out to make new connections.

I am on the teen board of Beyond Differences. Our main goal is to spread a national movement of educating and talking to mainly middle school students about social isolation. Kids open up and have insights into social isolation and bullying and share personal experiences to the point of tears. It reinforces my belief about what I heard in the song "People" from Funny Girl. We all need someone there for us. We all need someone.

~ Talia

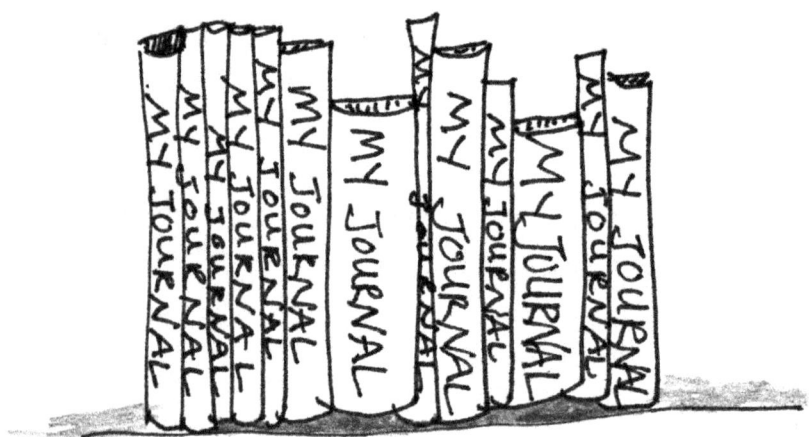

Chapter 5
A Sense of Peace

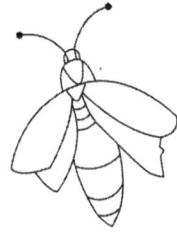

Alyssa & Pierre

I am not into sports, but I love to dance. I have been doing ballet since I was four years old and started jazz soon after. My mom is a cancer doctor, and my dad is a manager at a technology company. I have lived with a nanny my whole life, and she has been with my family for 18 years now.

~ Alyssa

My daughter was not into sports, either, but she did dance like you. She is 23, and just moved to Nashville to establish her independence! I grew up in Louisiana. My parents immigrated to the US from France after WWII. I was born four years later. I had a great chance to become fluent in French growing up, but my parents wanted to assimilate themselves into the language and culture of their new home so they only spoke French when they wanted to talk about something they didn't want me to understand. I met my wife when I was getting an MBA at Tulane. I like to tell people that she went to graduate school to get an education, and I went to find a wife!

My wife still works, but I am recently retired after qualifying for disability benefits. Although I have stage IV colorectal cancer, I have a good quality of life. I was diagnosed in 2004 and have already lived longer than statistics would suggest. At the time of my diagnosis, my daughter went on the internet and reported to me that I was only expected to live two years. I am glad to say that I have proven the internet wrong!

The good news is that the treatments are effectively arresting the cancer. For me, the name of the game is buying time until someday a cure for what I have will be found, but I am not real sanguine about that. Instead, my focus is to make each day count and being in my position does force me to focus on the more important things in life.

~ Pierre

I take dance at a school in the Mission called ODC. We recently had our winter concert at school, and I choreographed one dance and was in six dances which my friends choreographed. It was a lot of work but well worth it. It is so lucky that you have been able to fight off the cancer so well. How do you do it?

~ Alyssa

A woman I know who is battling stage IV lung cancer posted a quote to her website that I believe represents an important philosophy to live by. It is about not needing to know precisely what is happening, but to recognize the possibilities and challenges and to embrace the present moment with courage, faith and hope. I like to apply the "living in the moment" philosophy with a healthy dollop of humor in my life – just to keep things light and simple.

~ Pierre

I really enjoyed what you wrote, Pierre, and I am glad that you shared that with me. It is very inspirational because I feel pressured into thinking about what I want to do with my future when all I really want to do is focus on the present.

Now I dance every day of the week. I do ballet on Mondays, Tuesdays, and Fridays, a form of contemporary dance on Tuesdays and Thursdays, and another form on Sundays. I am going to try out for a summer intensive at my dance school, and I am very nervous.

~ Alyssa

I believe that finding something that you really, truly love to do can help one deal with just about anything. It is great that you have that sort of passion and commitment to dance. While money is important, it is not the most important thing in life. Health and happiness trump everything else. Follow your heart; the rest of you will find some way to keep up.

My treatments are going well, and the usual side effects have not yet reared themselves. My treatments continue every two weeks until April, and then I get a month off before my wife, daughter and I take a family vacation to South Africa and Botswana.

~ Pierre

I ended up getting into the summer dance intensive! I would love to dance professionally, but I don't think I could stand the intensity of competition. So, if dance doesn't work out, I would be interested in learning about the brain. For me, the next best thing to being a dance instructor would be to be a psychologist.

~ Alyssa

Congratulations! You are so lucky that dance means so much to you. I hope you always continue to find those things that make you happy. I get CT scans about every four to five months to assess the state of my tumors. This is probably the most anxious time for a cancer patient: waiting for the next report card. Alyssa, thank you so much for writing to me this year!

~ Pierre

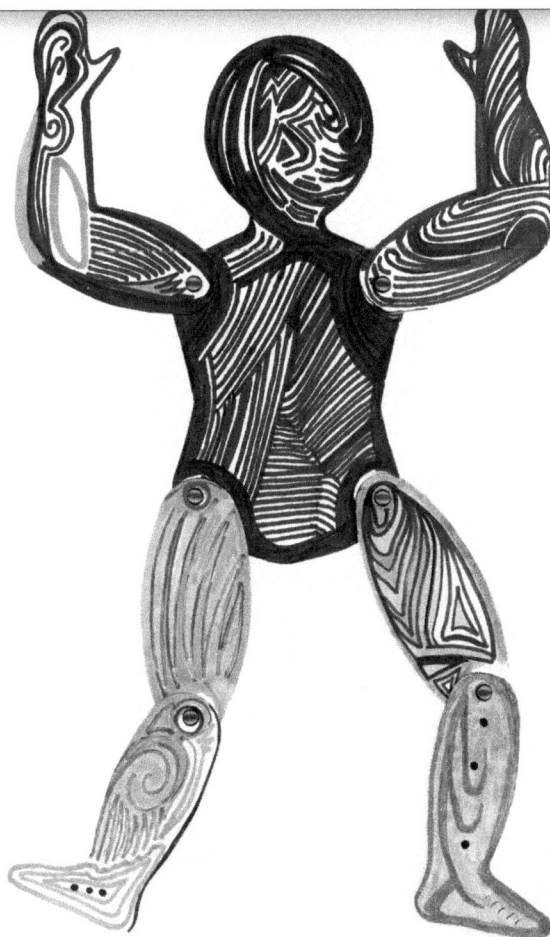

Cassidy & Bill

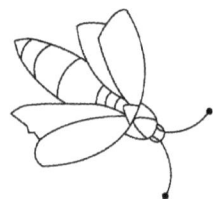

Right now I am playing tennis five days a week on my school's varsity tennis team, and I am hoping to be a captain next year. Other than tennis, I spend my free time this year tutoring underprivileged kids. My family consists of two brothers, a four-year-old German shorthaired pointer named Jeter (because my family consists of die-hard Yankee's fans), and a three-month-old kitten named Simba.

One reason I was especially interested in being your pen pal, is that I heard you are a Holocaust survivor. I cannot even begin to imagine. When I told my dad about you, he was especially touched as he was raised Jewish and even lived in Israel for parts of his childhood. I don't really practice a certain religion; my mom is Christian and we celebrate both Hanukkah and Christmas.

~ Cassidy

I feel being Jewish is being a member of a group. They are my people, and I feel at home amongst Jews. I have a nephew who went to medical school in Krakow where he married a Polish woman. Their children born here are both Christian and Jewish – no problem.

~ Bill

You said that you survived the war "by sheer luck." Do you ever think that there is a greater purpose for your survival? Sometimes, I can't help but believe that God has a reason for certain things, and maybe your survival was one of them? Were you in any danger when you moved to southern France? Or was it safer there?

Recently I have been going through a hard time. One of my good friends, who was only 16, died a few weeks ago. It feels so good to know that my kitty, Simba, is always there to curl up with me and hear me cry.

~ Cassidy

I am so sorry about your friend, Cassidy. This must be a difficult time for you. You must miss her terribly.

The fact that my family and I survived the Holocaust is, in my mind, no great design. It happened that we were in southwest France, not far from Toulouse; we hid in a small town where we were very obviously strangers to the locals. We were most afraid of a man who was an official, the local town crier. The French were under the control of the Germans who had many French do their dirty work.

Well, after the Germans were gone in 1944, we found out that the town crier was the head of the Resistance. When we asked him why did you not let us know, he answered: "I was undercover and could not reveal to you what I was." He also said he knew we were Jews, and he watched over us, and effectively we survived, untouched. My 64-year-old Grandfather, who lived in occupied Belgium, was picked up by the local police and taken to Auschwitz. He died in the cattle car on the way to a certain death, and he was a kind and generous and would not hurt a fly.

~ Bill

I am so sorry about your grandfather, but as you said, at the very least he didn't have to go through the horror of the camp. I can't even begin to imagine the bravery that is required to live through that. I am grateful that you had someone watching over you.

~ Cassidy

I belong to a French group, *Les Amis de la Culture Francaise*. We meet high school students that have a French program and engage them in conversation, and they are rated for their knowledge of French. The group awards cash prizes to the best students. It is not much cash, but we want to encourage them. *N'est-ce-pas?*

~ Bill

I, of course, agree that French is a beautiful language, and I am so glad you are reaching out to continue it. Cependant, je new sais pas si je serai capable de parler le Francais avec vous! Je vous promets, je ne peux pas parler tres bien. Au revoir, mon ami!

~ Cassidy

I love when you write to me in French; you are very good and should continue! Cassidy, I have hope for the future, and I am happy I survived the war so that I could write to a smart girl like you and my other pen pals. *Au revoir, ma gentile amie!*

~ Bill

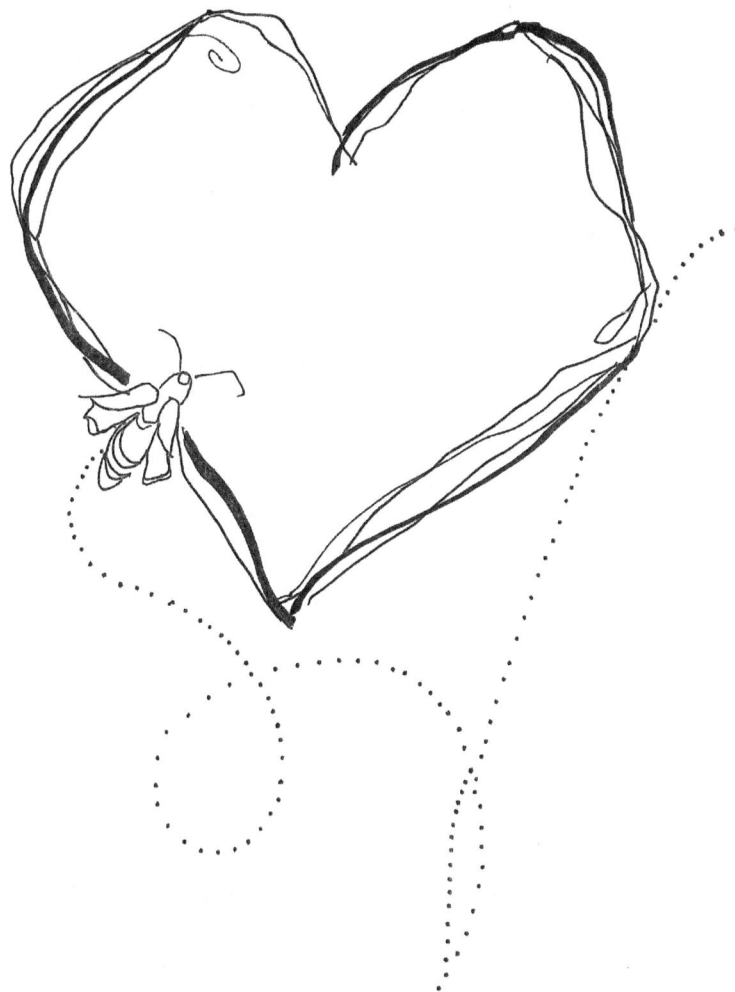

Haylee & Bill

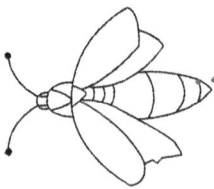

I am an elite gymnast and a soccer player. I have been doing gymnastics for 12 years, and I love it with a passion. I compete all over the world; it is very dangerous, and I have seen horrible things happen to people. I have seen injuries that can never be fixed and dreams crushed. I was offered to go big and make my dreams come true, but that meant no more high school. I decided that was not what I wanted.

One month ago, my good friend committed suicide. I cry myself to sleep almost every night. I love her more than anything. I would do anything to hear her voice just one last time. Her death will be on my mind every day, and it will affect me for the rest of my life. She has no idea how she has changed me. I will never be the same.

I understand that you were diagnosed with cancer, and I would like to know your condition. I have a lot of family members who have passed away from cancer; it was awful to experience every time, because I never saw it coming.

~ Haylee

I read your letter with concern. The fact that your friend killed herself recently is a big burden for a young person. I feel for you. There is something about your teenage friends that will stay with you forever. Believe me, I know; I am 86 years old now, so I have some experience.

I have had many operations as a result of my diagnosis of bladder cancer, but I still have my bladder. Others are not so lucky.

You made me think of soccer. When I was about ten years old and we were living on the coast of Belgium, the kids went to see a soccer match, but if it rained, we went to the movies. I prayed for rain. I did not like soccer, but I loved the movies.

~ Bill

I have been dealing and struggling every day with my friend's death. Since her death, I know of two other girls whom we have lost. High school has been too crazy for me. It is so hard. All of the homework, sports, loved ones lost; I have no idea how people get through it in one piece.

Your life seems full of obstacles and challenges, and I have no idea how you have overcome them. Did the war affect the way you view people now? My friend who died was Jewish. She and I planned a trip to Israel for our senior year – it kind of sucks that it isn't going to happen. I guess you never realize what you have until it is gone.

Cancer is so scary, not only for the one diagnosed, but also for their loved ones.

~ Haylee

I am so shocked that you have so many friends who have died, a moment of despair and they cannot face the problem. That is tragic. Life is wonderful. I enjoy my advanced years. I am 86 and still going strong!

I am making all the arrangements for my upcoming cruise next September. Cruises are great for seniors, but you would be bored. The food is so good that you can gain weight, but then you can go to the exercise rooms so you can pedal the calories away.

~ Bill

I am amazed by your life. You are a cancer survivor, WWII survivor, you are in your 80s and you are still going on cruises and living life to the fullest? I wish I could learn as much as I can from you.

Suicides are a horrible epidemic. I visit my friend's grave and just cry. I am trying my best to address the problem. I am starting a program at my school to help kids and educate them on depression so I can help them while helping myself. It has been pretty successful, and I have been satisfied with the success.

I can't wait to leave home and let my parents finally live on their own and even travel. They deserve that. My goal is to save up money, and when I get a job I will pay for my parents to go to Hawaii for two weeks.

~ Haylee

I can imagine you going to your friend's grave and crying; you must keep her in your heart, but you are young and have your whole lie ahead of you. Life is so wonderful; every day brings new things to see and do. My wife Harriet, died suddenly after 52 years of a good marriage. When something like this happens, some become very disturbed and cannot continue alone. I, on the other hand, felt that I have a few years left and I will make the best of it. In spite of my bladder cancer, in remission now, I do have a normal life and a lady friend in Florida as well!

~ Bill

Thank you, Bill. I think I am making a lot of progress moving past my friend's death. We are making progress together, and I realized that no matter what, she is never actually gone from me as I will always remember her.

~ Haylee

I hope your family knows what a treasure you are. I just had a medical check-up, and I am now cancer free for five years. You can never consider yourself cured. I am in remission, and must check again in a year and a half.

On May 26th, I turned 86. When you get old, you cling to family. Being alone is so sad, so many oldsters are alone. I am lucky. In spite of cancer, I can hear well and my eyesight is okay. "Count your blessings," I say to myself!

~ Bill

Whisper In My Soul

4

Letters exchanged between medical, nursing and pharmacy students
& adults coping with life-threatening illness

2011 ~ 2012

Chapter 1
Leap of Faith

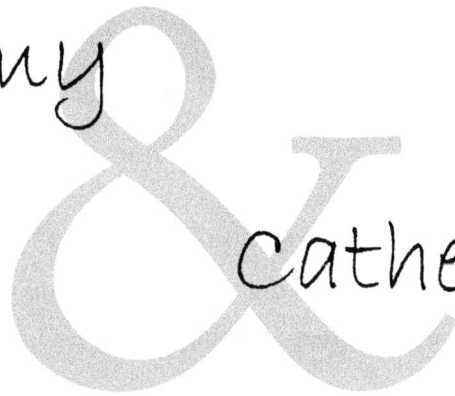

Amy & Catherine

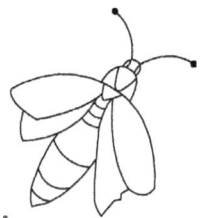

It is the last day of my ob/gyn rotation. I am a third-year med student, and after an exam on Friday, I will have my first vacation since mid-April last year. I have enclosed in my letter a little square for a quilt I am making. I am having a really hard time finding work/life balance; i.e., I have lots of work, but no life.

I have started a new life in a new apartment after a breakup, and I am trying to get to know myself and the quilt making project is all mine.

One of the reasons I wanted to do the Firefly Project was to collaborate with someone new, both by forming a friendship and by creating art. I also really miss getting letters. My grand mom used to write me often, but she died in 2009. She wrote letters to everyone, kept numerous journals, wrote essays about her life.

I also have many relatives with cancer, but have not talked to them much about it. What is your life like? I know that you have a dog, worked at Lucas film, have had lymphoma and breast cancer, but that's about it.

Amy

Sounds like you are making a beautiful quilt. Good luck finding your work/life balance, especially when you are on such a steep learning curve.

It is interesting to me that cancer touches so many people in so many different ways. I first got cancer in 1979. Cancer has been and continues to be a challenge for almost my entire adult life, for me, my husband and caregiver, and for our daughter. My breast cancer came from the life-saving new treatment at that time, full mantal radiation for the initial diagnosis of Hodgkins Lymphoma. Lucky for my daughter, it is not genetic.

How did your exam go, Amy?

Catherine

I am glad to hear that your cancer isn't genetic, although it must be frustrating to have it happen again. Was it different the second time?

My ob/gyn exam did go well. I got an evaluation that said I should speak up more. I am not shy, but I do find it difficult to be constantly thrust into new situations, and I like to observe before I jump in. I just finished my pediatrics rotation in Fresno. In some ways it was a big culture shock, but in other ways it seems like the culture of medicine can bridge those gaps, at least when I am at work.

~ Amy

I used to have a hard time speaking up, but then I was interviewing for an on air job on PBS, and there were three sections of the interview: written, spoken and on camera. I practiced in front of a still camera and made my husband be the audience. I got the job and overcame my shy speech in a big way.

I was 27 when I was first diagnosed and had never been sick. I was very frightened. When they first told me my tumor was malignant, I didn't put together that my malignant tumor could be cancer. When I did, it was a crystallizing moment for me. My daughter was three when I was diagnosed. It has been part of all our lives. I guess I am lucky that my husband of almost 38 years has stuck with me and has been a very stabilizing person in our daughter's life as I have had lots of radiation, chemo twice, multiple surgeries and am currently on a targeted therapy.

~ Catherine

The doctor I worked with today (I am on family medicine, which is all outpatient), made me sit up straight, speak loudly, and present without notes. It was tiring and surprisingly difficult; someday I will appear as competent as I am.

By the way, I was a very diligent child and dutifully followed PBS instructions to get my parents to donate every time – even when my dad explained that we had already donated!

I am 25 now and can't imagine being sick, Catherine, all of a sudden like you were. I wouldn't wish surgery or chemo on anyone.

~ Amy

Amy, I am sure you are competent or you would not have been able to sit up straight, with no notes and speak to your patients. I am sure they heard you!

~ Catherine

Your letters are a big treat for me. At first, I was not sure what to expect and not sure how to discuss cancer. But I have seen that illness and health affects our lives and influences our relationships in subtle ways too. We exist outside these experiences, but they are still there. Family medicine is done already, and I am more than halfway through my internal medicine rotation. I think I have finally hit my stride, and I think I want to go into this field.

~ Amy

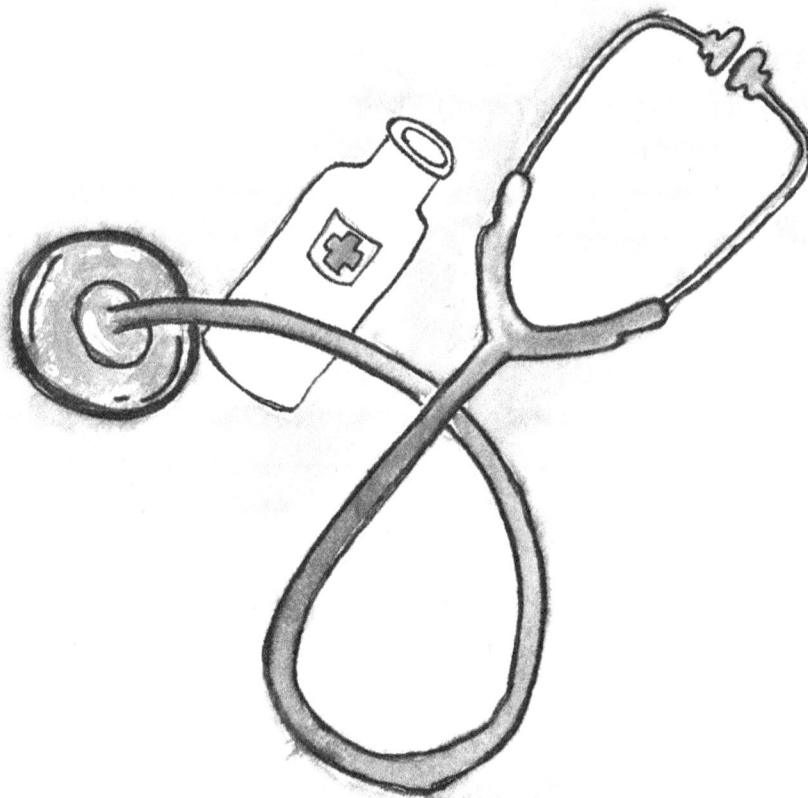

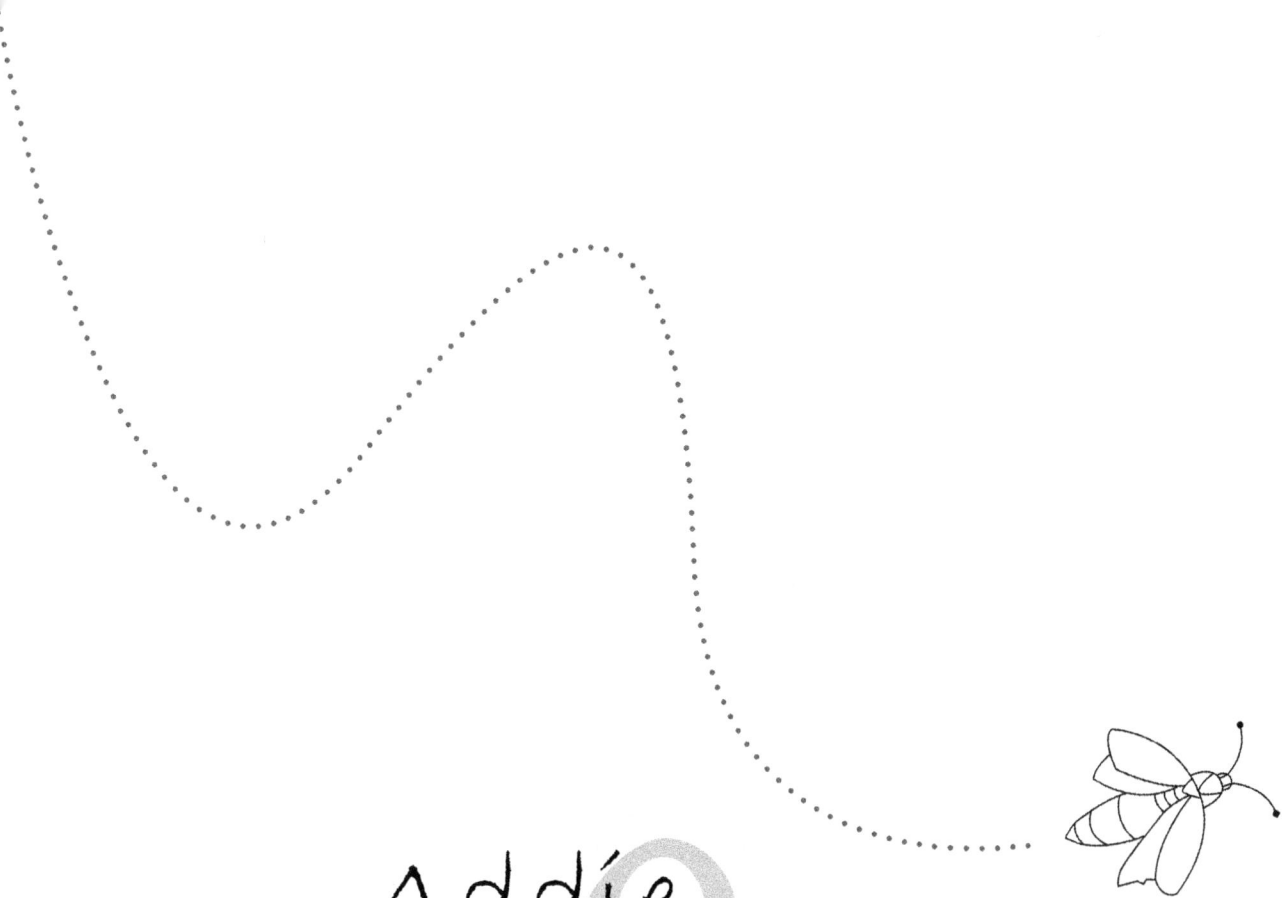

Addie & Janet

This is an unusual time for me, full of self-evaluation and waiting. I am applying to medical school, and I work at UCSF in breast cancer, assisting research projects and taking notes for patients who visit our clinic.

This is a big change for me. I worked for about five years after college as an NPR reporter before deciding in 2010 to become a doctor. I loved my prior career. Carrying a microphone helped me to pay attention to the important and beautiful qualities in people's voices and words and to feel connected to the landscapes I worked in and traveled through. I lived in Wyoming for three years and interviewed Peruvian sheepherders, oil workers, veterans with traumatic brain injury, and US Senators. I laughed and cried with strangers. I came to feel much more bound to the people I interviewed than to the thousands or millions listening to my stories. And so I decided to make a change. I left my reporting job, moved to Philadelphia and spent the academic year studying pre-medical sciences. Now that it is over, thank goodness, and I live in San Francisco in a vegetarian co-op with old friends from college, I am trying to find the strength to become the adult and the doctor I want to be. And, of course, being in my twenties, I have a bundle of doubts about whether I have made the right choice.

~ Addie

This is my second year participating in Firefly, and I believe it helped me so much last year to express myself and discuss things that sometimes I don't even talk about with some of my friends.

I am Japanese-American. I was born and raised in San Francisco. Went to college, moved back to San Francisco and worked in corporate America. One of my dreams was to live in New York, so I moved there and ended up working for Sesame Street. A few years later, I had a complete breakdown and moved back home. I didn't work for years and then my parents decided to open a restaurant. I ended up working there more than full time for years. Then my mother had a major stroke in 2008. I was her primary caregiver. In 2009 I was diagnosed with uterine cancer. Fertility was my biggest concern. They found more tumors. I got a full hysterectomy, and chemo. During that time my mother was also diagnosed with cancer and passed away in 2010.

Bravo for jumping ship! I think a lot of people are so fearful of doing that and later on in life, Addie, regret it or wonder where their hopes and dreams went. I don't think it is ever too late to start again. Ever!

~ Janet

I am typing this letter in San Antonio, at a breast cancer conference. You asked if it might be unnerving for me, not knowing whether I have made the right decision about leaving radio for medical school...you are so right. This conference makes me very aware of this: I can hardly understand what these people are saying! More daunting, I will not know for years whether I will be any good at medicine, or if I will enjoy it. Taking this leap felt fast and gutsy, but its after effects are emerging very slowly. I may not know for decades whether this was the right choice, and I will have to settle into that uncertainty.

Meanwhile – and this may just be my late 20s talking – other uncertainties are beginning to wear on me. I will be walking home from work, and I will catch myself thinking ridiculously existential thoughts. Am I enjoying my life? Why do I feel so tired recently? I know this sounds silly, but something powerful is changing inside me, an increasing sense that I have just one life, just this one, and that there is no way to do it right. I am working to quiet the questioning in order to focus on the joy of being alive, being healthy and able, having freedom of motion, but then, I don't know. Is asking big-picture questions about one's life helpful or just obsessive? I guess there are many ways to answer that question. Does this sound familiar to you?

~ Addie

I am really inspired by your leap of faith. It is always better to have tried than not to do it at all. I think you are very brave and no matter the outcome, you made the right decision.

For me, it is hard to be balanced and to not think too much when I have too many emotions. So sometimes, like now, the aftermath of cancer, infertility and my mom's death. . . too many emotions. I have had so much anxiety, that it was hard for me to leave the house.

I like to think of it as a volcano that just erupted. My doctor calls it dealing with a forest fire: first contain, then slowly put it out. He says I am still burning a little, but mostly embers.

I have learned to enjoy life, to enjoy both the little and big things. It is hard though, and sometimes I actually feel guilty for not being thankful and happy. I have also learned there is nothing I can do about things I can't control, but I can control how I choose to deal with the cards I have been dealt.

I still have a hard time with not being able to bear children. I know there are other ways to be a mom, but I am still grieving and find myself asking God "Why?" I think, for me, knowing that I won't be able to naturally have kids is just as upsetting as hearing I have cancer.

~ Janet

I feel pain in my chest as I read your letters. Both of the sources of your grief have to do with motherhood, and I imagine your feelings about each loss may be somewhat intertwined. My mom and I are extremely close: I am an only child raised by my mom alone. I really struggle with the possibility of losing her. I often wonder if there is something I can do now, something I can do better to be better to her. What I hope for you is that you will find peace in your grief and courage to live fully in the many ways open to you still.

~ Addie

I never felt close to either of my parents growing up. They didn't have that much time for me as they were busy running the restaurant. They also had a pretty rocky marriage, and I was angry at them for not making enough time for me. But recently I have been talking to my father, and he has been sharing a lot more about his youth, and my mom's, so I can understand where they came from. They were both raised in rural Japan, moved to America with nothing in their pockets and became working middle class, putting two kids through private school, owning a home and running a successful business. I am learning to appreciate and respect them both.

One thing I wish I could have done with and for my mom was to tell her and show her how much I loved her while she was healthy. Although she was still able to speak after her stroke, she did have quite a bit of brain damage. I am so thankful, even though I wished she didn't have to go through the pain, but at the end I had the time and chance to tell her everything I wanted. We were actually able to say the words "I forgive you" to each other. I know she and my father did their very best to raise me, and they know I am doing my best to be a good daughter and a good person.

~ Janet

How much did you know about your parents' background when you were growing up? Do you think that if you had known more you might have found forgiveness earlier on?

I love, love, love your letters. I want you to know how grateful I am for your openness and warmth. You have a big, shining spirit, and I have no doubt that anything you set your mind to in life will happen for you.

~ Addie

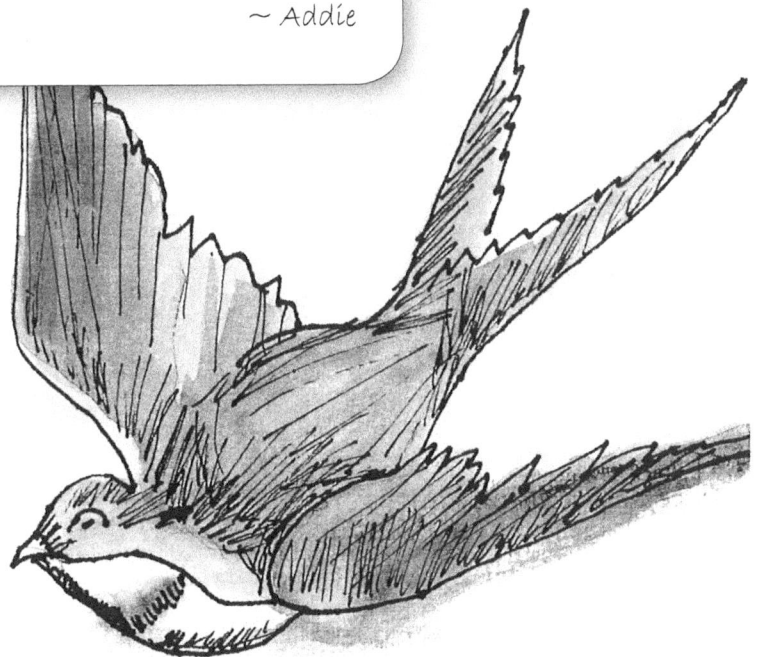

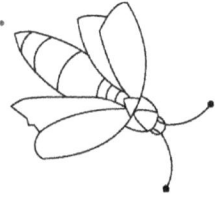

Nichole & Janet

I was born in Taiwan and immigrated to the US when I was seven years old. I was raised by my aunt and uncle in Fremont, California. I still keep in touch with my parents in Taiwan, so I still feel close to my Taiwanese heritage and culture. I went to UC Berkeley, and I always wanted to be a lawyer. While an undergrad, I started an organization called Saving Mothers, which is still a big part of my life today. I fell in love with public health, especially maternal health, and it was my love of this that led me to medical school.

Now that I am a second-year medical student, my love for women's health has grown, and I am excited to learn more. I find almost any subject fascinating and truly feel fortunate to be where I am at this moment in my life.

~ Nichole

Is medical school like you expected? Does having your public health background give you a different perspective on medicine? Why did you move to the US?

I was diagnosed with uterine cancer. I had a conservative surgery to keep me fertile. They thought I had uterine cancer stage I and borderline ovarian cancer. Then they found more tumors so I had a full hysterectomy – turns out I have a very strange cancer – something my oncologist and pathologist have never seen. So I am now stage IIIC.

Right now I teach abacus once a week. I used to practice when I was younger. Some of my students are better than my current rusty level, but I can still teach them!

~ Janet

I love medical school. I think my public health background and my travels give me a different perspective. I am still deciding what kind of medicine I want to practice. I am naturally inclined to be an ob/gyn, but I want to keep my options open.

I started Saving Mothers after I did my thesis on misoprustal and maternal death. We now send ob/gyn residents and nurses to provide care, as the goal is to have public health projects and training programs that will help providers in Guatemala and Liberia better serve the women in their communities.

It breaks my heart that you had to go through the cancer treatments. As a woman, I can understand a little about your feelings toward the hysterectomy. Have you thought about adoption? Coming from a background where I was raised and legally adopted by my aunt and uncle, I think it can be extremely fulfilling. My aunt and I are very close, and she is the person I love most in the world. I decided a long time ago that I want to adopt at some point in my life.

~ Nichole

I am having such a hard time grieving infertility that I have a hard time even looking at babies. It is the bearing more than the genes. I want to experience pregnancy and birth and that physical bond that is a gift that we women receive when we are born.

I can't even begin to imagine the pressures and time management issues. When do you have to decide what specialty you will practice? And, right now, I can't believe that you were able to find the time to write to me!

~ Janet

So this week, I am trying very hard to try to get a good third-year rotation schedule. It is good and bad that UCSF has so many hospitals where you can do these rotations. After medical school you have residency which is when you actually start having real responsibilities in taking care of the patient. As medical students we are at the bottom of the totem pole.

Thank you for sharing all that you have. I really don't think that this would have worked without your brutal honesty and taking a leap of faith in each other. Thank you for taking the plunge with me.

~ Nichole

Matt & Suzanne

I just graduated from Princeton last May and transplanted myself to San Francisco in July. I have lived in New Jersey my whole life. If you have ever come across the show "Jersey Shore," then you've unfortunately seen some of the more embarrassing parts of my home town. I am interning at UCSF while I apply to medical school. We are testing several new drugs in hopes of developing more effective chemotherapy treatments.

~ Matt

I am 49 years old. This is significant as my own mother never made it to this age. She died seventeen days before her 49th birthday from breast cancer, I was 16 at the time. This October, 17 days before my 49th year, I took time to reflect about my mother and my life. The next morning, I awoke feeling energized knowing that I have lived past the age that she had died. I knew in my bones that her life and my life and journey are different. This is significant because I was diagnosed with stage IV breast cancer to bone only after a first diagnosis in 2008. In this letter I will introduce myself to give you a small idea of who I am.

I was married when I was 43, first marriage for both of us. I married a good man. I have a 29-year-old daughter. I had her when I was 19. I raised her alone. She is tall with red hair and brown eyes. My daughter and I grew up together. We speak daily.

My mother introduced me to health foods. I remember drinking apple cider vinegar and water for your blood when I was 12, fresh juices when I was 15, no white sugar products starting at 15. After her death I became a vegetarian and became conscious of the foods I ate.

~ Suzanne

I hear our physicians emphasizing the importance of a healthy diet to patients all the time. Doctors need to advocate for better health habits on the part of their patients, not just when problems arise.

I interact with breast cancer patients almost every day. It has been a powerful, humbling, and inspiring experience meeting women who are facing such formidable challenges; I truly admire the courage that you and others must have in order to deal with such a difficult disease.

~ Matt

For weeks after my second surgery, I felt better than I had ever felt in my life. I have been a strong and healthy woman all my life, but this was different. Then radiation started, and everything changed. I felt like my soul was being sucked out of me. I cried for the first week and each and every day I went to get the treatments. I was exhausted and could not understand that this was the way cancer is treated in the 21st Century. At three weeks, I stopped my treatments. I was supposed to do six weeks but just could not continue.

A year later, the breast cancer was back and in parts of my bones. From this point forward my life changed. I realized in my body that I could die. I wept deeply, and as I did that everything that I was resisting, feeling sadness about, and everything that was tied to the past washed away. I had broken wide open.

I am participating in a study called "The Lilac Study." They are studying emotions in people with advanced cancer. The studies have shown people with more positive emotions in their lives go on to live longer, are healthier and feel more satisfied with life. I hope all the doctors at UCSF will be able to read this study and incorporate it into their way of being with patients.

~ Suzanne

I am reminded of my grandmother's strength during her own battle with advanced lung cancer. Her lesson to me was to always keep perspective on things in life, and that is a lesson that hasn't left me since. Despite the fact that she was always able to maintain a composed exterior, I can only imagine what she must have felt on the inside, and I sincerely wish that she'd been able to receive the extraordinary quality of cancer care and support that I see patients receive here every week.

My experiences here at UCSF have made me strongly consider oncology as the field I want to pursue. My time with my grandmother provided much of the underlying motivation for my pursuit of a career in medicine.

~ Matt

Cancer can be a scary diagnosis. There is a lot of fear around it especially since the term "there is a war on cancer" has been coined. Who wants to relate to what is going on inside their body as a war? What I have learned from those with cancer is that they are afraid to get diagnosed because of their fears about cancer, and because they are terrified of the treatments. My second diagnosis of metastasized breast cancer has changed my life. One of the big things that changed is fear. I was constantly on the go, keeping busy and having the feeling of not having enough time. Now I am more at ease and trusting. I feel more connected and in tune with life.

I am putting myself first now. I did not do that before. So now, here I am with a second diagnosis like my mother, at the same age. I know that something has to change for me to live.

No matter what type of medicine you decide to specialize in, your openness and finding value in relating to patients will bring so much to them. You could end up being a leader in integrative oncology. Bless your grandmother for her influence in so many ways.

~ Suzanne

While I meet new people routinely through my job, Suzanne, and even get to hear their deepest concerns before and during their appointments, it is rare that I get to have such a meaningful dialogue and truly see a complete picture of someone's journey as I have with you. Thank you so much.

~ Matt

My test results all look good, and the tumor is shrinking. That is all good to hear. I did have some bumps on my breast that my doctor said were metastasized bumps. It made me sad for a bit. They were a reminder that I have cancer. Most of the time I live my life giving appreciation for so much. But moments like seeing the bumps and knowing what they are can bring tears to my eyes. Then I take several big breaths and close my eyes to really feel it in my body and release it. Life goes on, and each moment I have a choice.

Thank you for taking the time to participate in Firefly. You have inspired me and imprinted hope on my journey to restore the idea of treating the whole person when dealing with cancer.

~ Suzanne

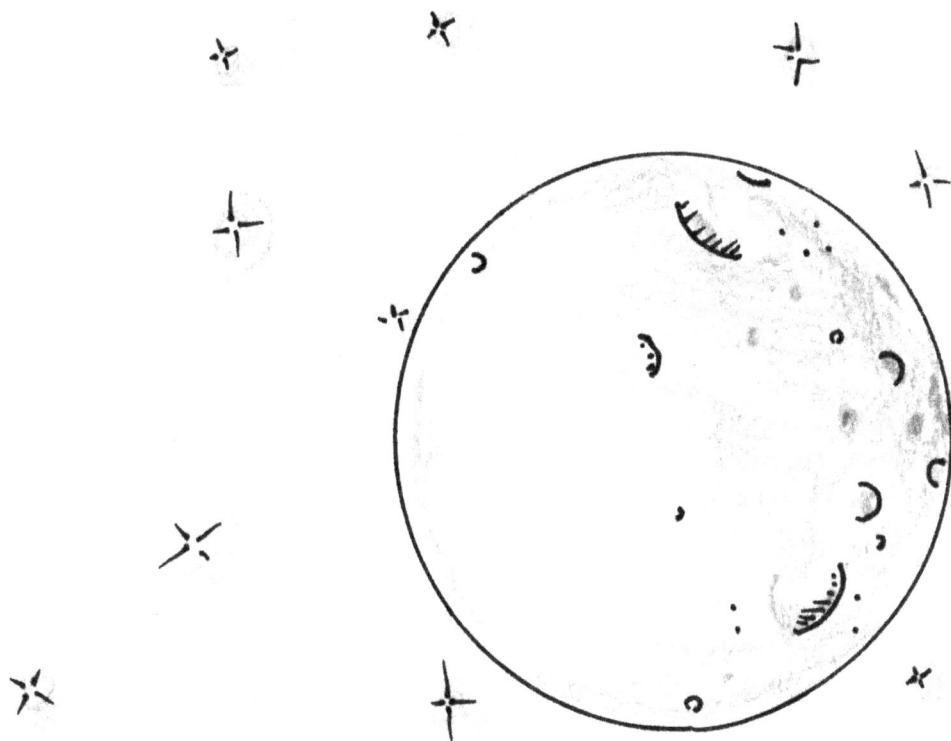

Chapter 2

A Deliberate Life

Brittany 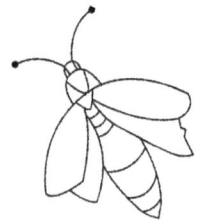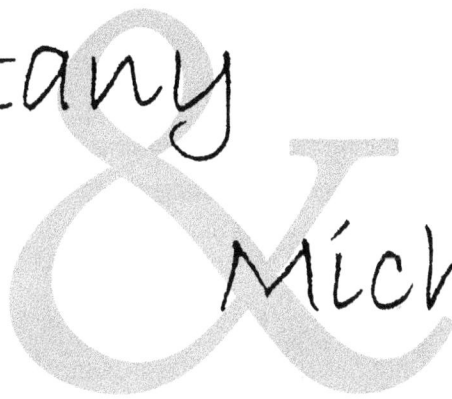 Michelle

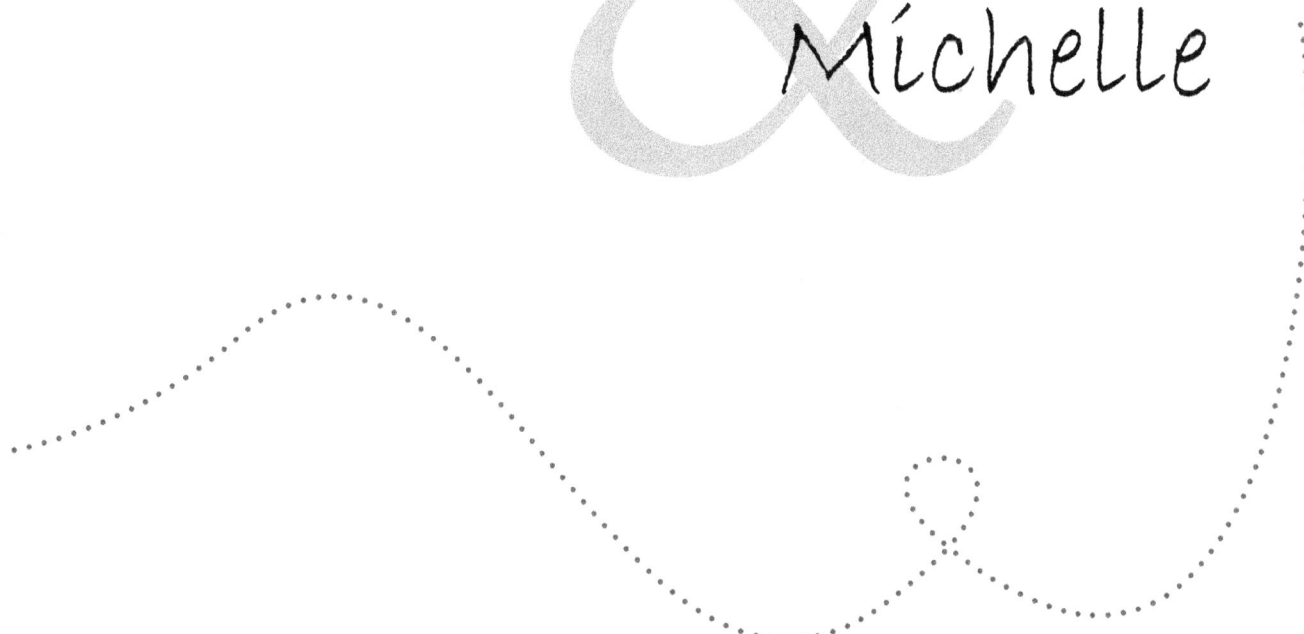

On January 1st, 2010, when I was living in LA and working in public relations and the entertainment industry, I made a New Year's Resolution: I would make moves toward pursing what I knew I always wanted to do: be a doctor. I quit my job in LA, moved to Philadelphia to complete a rigorous year of post-baccalaureate pre-med science classes. In other words, I went through pre-med boot camp.

Doctoring has always been on my mind. My father is a doctor and my mother is an aerobic dance instructor, so I grew up in a household that talked a lot about health.

I loved that you hired a private investigator to reunite with the love of your life. I am a pre-med intern, and the best part of my job is interacting with patients.

~ Brittany

I am 71 years old, and it still boggles my mind every time I either say that or put it down on paper because I don't feel that age at all. I, too, always loved medicine, but when I was growing up, women weren't encouraged to become doctors. I was told I could be a good nurse or a teacher, and I didn't want to do either.

The opportunities that women have now to pursue their life long dreams are amazing. Sometimes I regret that I did not become a physician, but my path has been rewarding in and of itself.

Yes, I was reunited with my first love in 1996, Brittany. We will be celebrating our 15th wedding anniversary. I did hire a private detective to find him, and he was looking for me on the internet at the same time. It was right after we discovered each other that I was diagnosed with breast cancer. My husband arranged for me to be seen at UCSF. I had a brand new job, and the day I started it, I also started radiation.

Fast forward to 2005 when I retired and was diagnosed once again, this time on the other breast! Being a cancer survivor has given me a very different perspective on life. My priorities are much different and I don't allow the small stuff to crowd my thoughts.

I was thinking about something that means a great deal to me, Brittany. My mother, as she grew older, used to tell me about how she was treated by medical practitioners as she aged. She said that a good portion of them talked to her as if she was a senile old fool. She was anything but! As I am growing older, I seem to be encountering the same thing. It is very demeaning and demoralizing, and I think it is important that the medical community be sensitive to this issue. I believe that dignity and respect should be given to each patient.

~ Michelle

There is a lot of emphasis in the medical field on improving doctor/patient communication. You are right, patients deserve to be treated as more than just their age. How many years old you are doesn't indicate that one's intelligence is declining; rather it should indicate that the person has been with their own body for that many years, and they know their body best.

You hired a private detective to find your husband? Tell me more!

~ Brittany

Well, my husband and I first met when I was 19 and he was 24 and just out of college. We were set up on a blind date by a mutual friend. We dated for a couple of years, and then he decided to leave Philadelphia.

We both married other people. I was married for 25 years, got both an undergrad and master's degree and then divorced my husband. I decided to find my "old flame" and hired a detective to do that. He found him, I called him, and we have been together ever since. My husband was right in San Rafael, and when I called him, the first thing he said to me, after he caught his breath, was, "How did you know I was looking for you?" And the rest, as they say, is history. He has stood by me through every procedure and is my champion.

I am so happy that I have had a chance to correspond with you. You have a fantastic attitude, and I know you are really good at what you do.

~ Michelle

I attended a breast cancer conference in Vienna, Austria. It didn't matter where the attendees came from, or what language they spoke; they were experts in the field of breast cancer coming together with a common goal; to share and learn.

~ Brittany

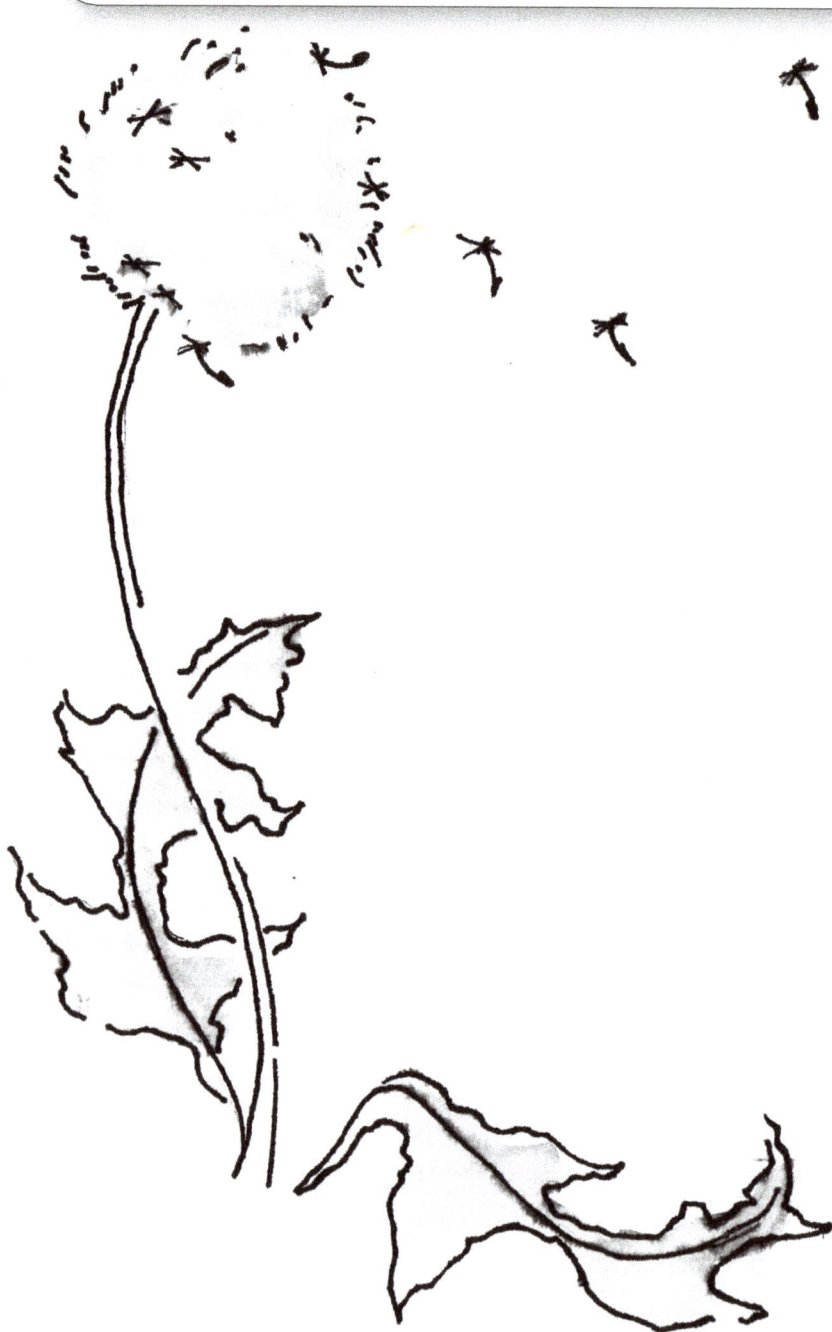

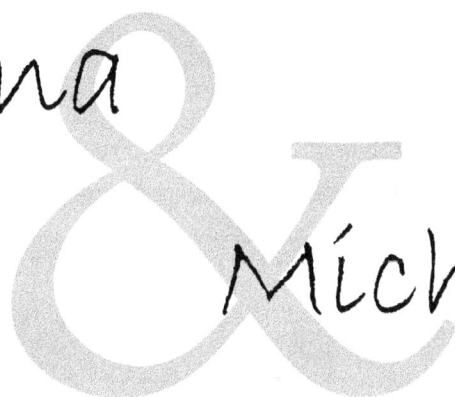

Tina & Michelle

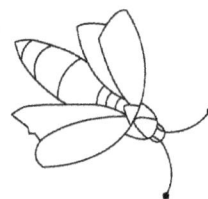

I am 28 years old yet many regard me as an "old soul." Perhaps it is the serious demeanor and my introverted nature; or because I am the oldest of four and needed to be responsible at a relatively young age. Sometimes I feel that my siblings are my children; I do not mean that there is a sense of ownership, rather responsibility and protectiveness that I have for them.

I am in an accelerated nursing program. This is my second bachelor's degree, but I finally feel like I have found something that I would love to do for the rest of my life. I want to specialize in oncology and teach down the line to pass on my knowledge. I come into this Firefly program with an open mind and an open heart.

~ Tina

> I went back to school as an adult and completed a Bachelor's and a Master's degree. I was married at the time, had two daughters, ran a house, driving carpools, and studying all the time. I had a purpose and never lost track of what it was.
>
> I have had both surgery and radiation for breast cancer, and I am now cancer-free. My priorities are so much different now. I see my friends anguishing over stuff that in the scheme of things, is very inconsequential.
>
> ~ Michelle

Congratulations on being a cancer survivor! I cannot imagine how enduring breast cancer twice must have affected you and your loved ones. Did you have any negative experiences? I hope you were able to keep a journal, photos or some sort of record of "you" throughout these times. Sometimes we may feel that our stories are only significant to us, but in actuality, our experiences, captured in pictures, writing or art can help everyone understand us better.

I do not know if nursing school has changed me, but more than anything else, the nursing program enabled me to acknowledge and address my personal biases and misconceptions about others, about life. Having the capacity to empathize and think beyond my own bubble, so to speak, has revitalized my vision of life.

Simultaneously I sometimes wonder if I am experiencing a slight disconnect with some friends who are unable to reflect beyond their own lives.

I graduated! It is just now settling in that I am done with the program. I even woke up in a panic one morning because I dreamt that I had missed an exam.

I am the first generation to be born in the United States. Both of my parents are from Vietnam. Being the oldest child and a daughter meant that I needed to be a role model for my siblings and, at times, a second mother to them. My siblings and I were born in Napa, famous for the vineyards, but it was a small town then that was predominantly Caucasian. Our holidays were a mixture of Vietnamese and American food. As children, we did not understand why our father was so against McDonald's; we wanted anything and everything American.

~ Tina

I did not keep a journal during my experiences going through diagnosis and treatment as I have an aversion to committing my personal thoughts to paper, and I didn't want to risk being criticized. However, after reading your paragraph about how it could help those who come after, I think I have changed my mind.

You asked about my negative experiences. There were two physicians that I fired because of their demeanor. They weren't a good fit for an ongoing relationship, so I requested someone else. I do remember reacting to a group that was called "Y Me" a cancer support group. I would never belong to any group with a name like that; it plays into victimhood. My answer is "Why Not Me?" Illness can strike anyone.

~ Michelle

I am happy to say that I passed my exam and received my nursing license! I cried a little bit when I found out, not only because I found a career that I love, but because this represents and means so much more to me than just a job. A weight has been lifted off my shoulders because I finally feel that I will have the means to support my parents as they age.

I want to make sure that my parents can depend on me in the future. I figure that this is the least I can do for all that they have done for, and given to, me.

It is difficult for a new grad to get a job. Most places are only looking to hire experienced nurses. One of the things I have learned from my parents is that there is nothing wrong with starting at the bottom and working your way up!

~ Tina

Congratulations! I feel it in my bones that you will find a job soon!

~ Michelle

Death is such a sensitive topic, but sometimes I disagree with the way we approach it with such fear or even disdain – until WE are forced to face it. All of us will face it sooner or later. Perhaps we can develop a deeper appreciation for the opportunities we are given and the memories we have.

~ Tina

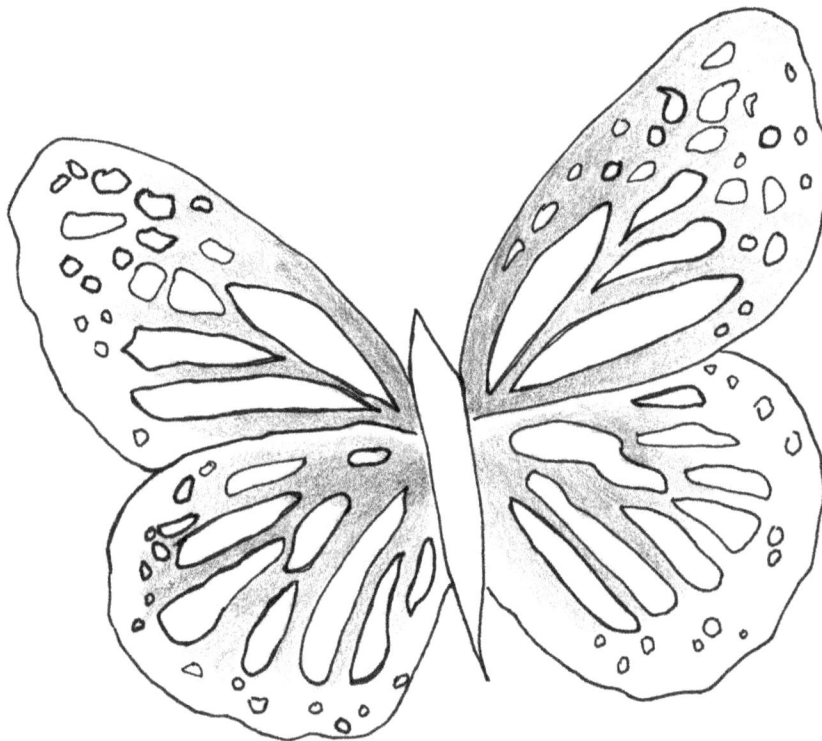

Jay & Hannah

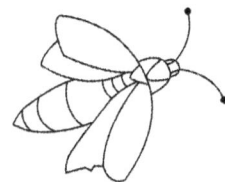

It feels like a long time since we exchanged letters within the Firefly Project a few years ago. You were writing about your experience during treatment for breast cancer, and I was writing about my mom's encounter with breast cancer. At the time, I had not really spoken with my mom about that since her aggressive and successful treatment.

A lot has happened on my end since then, and I am sure on yours as well. I matriculated at the Columbia College of Physicians and Surgeons, but decided to take a leave of absence. Then I had some misgivings about returning to NYC for the next four years. I found New York cramped and unpleasant, especially since a lot of my hobbies: mountain biking, surfing, hiking, are harder to do there. This made me question my desire to become a doctor after all.

Things were clarified for me when my girlfriend had a sudden, unprovoked cardiac arrest two months before I was due to return to Columbia. It was surreal as she is an athletic 24-year-old with no family history of heart problems. Lucky doesn't begin to describe how she avoided brain or other permanent damage. I choose not to matriculate.

I am now living back in San Francisco with my girlfriend. I have applied to California medical schools. I am also working for an exciting start-up company in Palo Alto, which is unlike anything I have ever done.

~Jay

I can't tell you how glad I am to be writing to you again! Based on your experiences in the past year, you too have been through a critical time that has allowed you to look differently at life. Does it bring wisdom?

Here it is 31 months after my diagnosis, and I am starting to feel numb. I am annoyed at the driver who moves from lane to lane without the considerate blinker. I am yelling at my kids for not picking up the dog poo in the backyard quickly enough to prevent its traction throughout the house. I am looking at my friends with annoyance at their trivialities and negative energy. I prefer being raw. I liked feeling every emotion and then a few.

I liked fighting to preserve my life, as it made life tangible. It made good sense and made me feel whole, a part of something bigger.

I am interested in knowing how you feel on the level that makes you alive. Is there a switch that can be activated? I have a lot of friends who have been diagnosed with recuring cancers, mostly breast cancers and a few brain tumors. I wonder as I watch them battle or decide to surrender: am I next? If I am, am I living a "deliberate life?" Am I choosing my course or is it being chosen for me?

~ Hannah

It is funny, the delay between letters sent in the mail. I am so used to the instant message, all interactions on a whim. So I like how this helps us step back and survey, to exercise a longer form of thinking and writing.

I imagine we are in a dusty old library full of obsolete paper books but also quiet and separate from the swirling chaos outside, and the books span the ages. Out of the window are passing seasons, not days; time unwinds so we can see its full expanse. Thanks for bringing me back here.

I certainly feel wiser, but to call myself wise so soon after escaping such foolish habits of thought which really had me trapped couldn't be true. I am certainly more peaceful and content with myself. I am just getting back on the road to wisdom and knowledge, a never-ending one for sure. Whenever I hear that word, wisdom, I think of the Socrates quote about the wise man understanding just how much he doesn't know.

I can relate to suddenly feeling less of a purpose, probably to an even greater extent when I left Columbia and what I'd grown to believe was my only shot at a meaningful life. I felt at times like things could only get worse for me and the people I love. I saw a future unfurl that was worse than hopeless, which no one else could yet see. But making a commitment to continue to try towards something better, outside of myself, and to not put too much faith in my powers of prediction, helped make the difference. I prefer acceptance to surrender.

When I sit down to write to you, there is a sense of freedom I experience, a letting go of any sort of judgment; it is like being in the cloud where things just are.

I still have the scars and fear the worst on occasion, but I have had a certain amount of distance and feel less inclined to continue to pursue that psychological war. I have let the feelings wash through me. I don't carry them around anymore. They are not who I choose to be right now. I also realize, as it sounds like you do, that the sense of optimism and immunity could change at the drop of a hat, or the reading of a CT, PET or MRI.

My purpose, at the moment, is cancer related both professionally and as a volunteer. It is not, however, my identity. Time has shifted, and I have found ground under my feet. It did not happen overnight. And I know too well that, as you have said, the cloud of darkness could easily shade the sun. However, the fear is less, and I hope to start moving more slowly and deliberately.

Perhaps there are a few stages of grief in illness; I am now at one end. You, my kind gentle soul, are at the other end of the journey. It is a fragile place, but one where you have the opportunity to learn much about yourself, others and the world around you.

~ Hannah

I have thought a lot about living a life of balance since Columbia University, Hannah. I take more care than I would have before to protect time with family and friends, and to do things I love. I am also deciding what I want to do, maybe eventually what specialty to go into. I am convinced that medicine is one thing that I could be passionate about, and it is what I want to do.

My girlfriend has been studying and stressing a lot about the Boards. She is doing fine now. You do give up a lot of freedom going into medicine; this is the test that determines residency choices. Despite the stress, she keeps it all in perspective. We're always happy when she has some down time and we can cook a meal or go for a run together, and we are planning a vacation for afterwards as a light at the end of the tunnel.

~Jay

My breast cancer diagnosis three-year anniversary is a few days away. It seems so distant. Another time, another place, and yet, I know my separation from sickness could elude me. It could come screaming in my ear or whisper in my soul and stop my breath.

I am also turning 50 in a few short weeks. I am sure that seems old to you, Jay. Hell, it seems OLD to me. The knowledge attained by 50 is overwhelming. Perhaps you have to make all the mistakes necessary to get to this place. It is a place filled with confidence, assuredness and calm.

Gratitude is something I have been thinking about. When you are first diagnosed, you think about it often. As time goes by, you think about it less and take more for granted. I don't feel as grateful or as emotionally raw. What is it that I was to have learned from the journey of the past three years? What is supposed to stay with me, grow and change me? Make me better or worse as a person? Understand and appreciate the value and worth of this life?

~ Hannah

I had my 25th birthday at the end of April. Half of 50 must seem pretty young to you too. Age is just a number, but also a natural yard post for where we are relative to where we want to be and where we are going.

You have a spirit that burns bright and young, regardless of numbers. And I think the wisdom you carry, your calm assuredness, means that you are mostly sailing a course that needs only subtle input and adjustment.

Happy Birthday, Hannah. I am grateful to have had this opportunity to reflect with you deeply about things that really matter. And, of course, your three-year anniversary from that diagnosis has become an important part of your life story, but one that does not menace as nastily, and from which you will be able to draw strength in the future.

~ Jay

Having lived half my lifetime, you seem so accomplished and wise! Life goes by faster now; it is as if the world is hurling by. Each year comes with a comfort, an elasticity, taking a new shape all its own. For me, it is MY shape. Mine alone, taking others into consideration, but I can say with confidence, it truly is MY life now.

~ Hannah

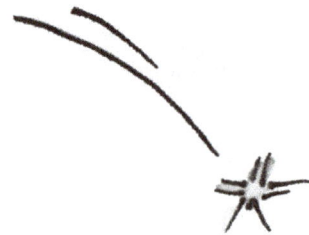

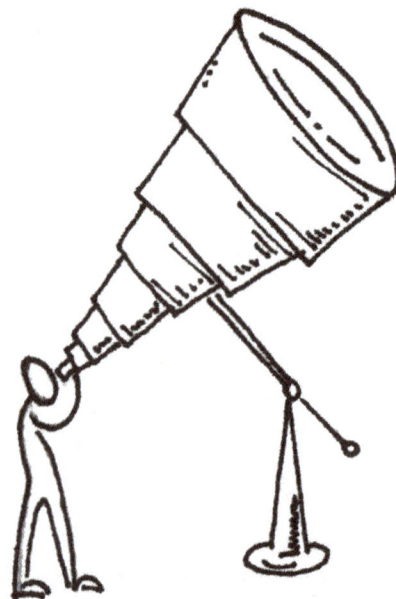

Melinda & Joan

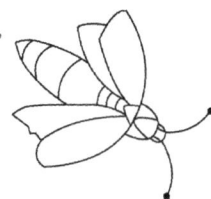

Currently I am second-year pharmacy student. It has been quite a roller coaster experience for me. The curriculum and responsibilities have been much tougher than I expected. There are times when I love everything I am learning and days when I feel absolutely overwhelmed and homesick. Well, only three more years to go!

During my first year of pharmacy school, I definitely spent too much time indoors studying and not enough time exploring, so this year I decided to take in more of my surroundings.

I learned about this Firefly Project through an elective offered at my school. The idea of having this chance to communicate with another person in such a meaningful way greatly appealed to me. I would be honored if you would be willing to share your experiences with me regarding your condition.

~ Melinda

I have an amazing 13-year-old daughter. I have been alone with her since she was three. I met her father while traveling through Indonesia in 1997. He is Balinese, and we lived together in San Francisco with Emma and then decided it was best to separate. He moved back to Bali; I have taken Emma there four times as we love the Hindu culture.

In 2008, I was diagnosed with breast cancer. The whole world stopped for me that day. I couldn't imagine not being here with my daughter. After nearly a year, I was finished with treatment. I am now taking a drug for five years to help keep it from coming back. It is always in the back of my mind though.

~ Joan

I can only imagine, and it probably pales in comparison, how you must have felt upon hearing the news that you had breast cancer. I am glad that your daughter was by your side throughout the whole ordeal. Your daughter Emma sounds absolutely lovely; it is great that you two are so close.

~ Melinda

For Thanksgiving, Emma and I prepared a feast and drove to Sacramento to visit my mother who was in the hospital. She has been very sick the last year first with breast cancer, then recently with a broken pelvis. I served our dinner out of a cooler in the hallway of the hospital. Something I am coming to terms with is the fact that my mother will probably pass in the next year. I think I am accepting of it, but there sure has been a lot of family drama around it. It has been very stressful.

We are trying to get our ticket to Bali. Emma will do her "Tooth Filing" ceremony with her cousins. This is a purification where they file her eye teeth. In the Balinese belief system, the ceremony helps people rid themselves of the invisible forces of evil. Teeth are the symbol of lust, greed, anger, insobriety, confusion and jealousy. Filing the teeth, therefore, renders someone both more physically and more spiritually beautiful, as well as symbolizing the rite of passage for an adolescent into adulthood. I hope she is ready for this!

~ Joan

The Tooth Filing ceremony sounds very interesting. I have never heard of anything quite like it before. Do you know if it is painful at all?

During Spring Break I went to New York. I have never been. It is incredible how we were walking around at 4:00 am, and the streets were still crowded. Five days is too short a trip, and now it is back to school I go. And, unfortunately, my resolution to get more sleep went out the window last quarter; it was pretty much impossible during finals week.

~ Melinda

My heart is broken as my mother died on May 11th.

Losing my mother is harder than I realized.

~ Joan

Alyse & Kate

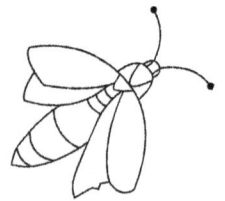

I moved here in July to start working as a pre-medical intern at the Breast Care Center. I play the violin (classical music). When I was a teenager I wanted to be a professional violinist, but later in college, I decided that I wanted to become a doctor. I haven't settled into a rhythm yet where I can play my violin every day. Instead, I have been trying all these new things: taking a boxing class, taking part in conversation exchanges where I meet Spanish speaking people to practice English and Spanish conversations (a bit like a dating service)... and then there is work.

~ Alyse

I have actually been delayed in starting this letter because I found a new lump in my breast, and even though I know that this is most likely scar tissue or something else, I can't get out of the emotional tailspin until someone official says it is not cancer. Just so you know how crazy the whole thing is, I have had a bilateral mastectomy, so the probability is pretty low that this is a new tumor, but all I can think about is how the last time I found something like this, my life totally changed. Maybe it is PTSD. Like I said, part of the craziness of this disease is learning to live with it and also trying to find a balance when sometimes a lot of the time I am just scared. I am 35 years old, a stage IV cancer patient, which means that I will be on chemo for the rest of my life.

I have always loved music too. I find that singing especially is a huge emotional release, and my challenge is to try to convey the full emotion that I am feeling into a song. Last year I tried out for X Factor in Los Angeles because I was so angry about my lung surgery and the fact that I thought it might affect my singing. I didn't make the final cut for the live show tryouts, but I was in the last group before that, which was 450 out of 13,000 so that felt pretty good six weeks after lung surgery. I am going to try out again this year. Why not?

I absolutely love the strings. I play the piano so I have the sustain pedal but it is not the same, I can't crescendo on a sustained note on a percussive instrument, plus you guys just get great attacks that the piano just doesn't have. Right now the rhythm of my days is pretty much defined by chemo runs. I am on chemo one week and off the next.

Totally impossibly great news, Alyse! As it turns out, it looks like the lump that was in my breast is just scar tissue from my breast reconstruction after my mastectomy. So that takes a lot off of my mind. One of the hardest things about cancer is trying to come up with defense mechanisms to deal with the scares that come up and to keep moving even when sometimes you feel completely overwhelmed by fear. Anyway it is good that this scare appears to be nothing. But that just shows me that I need to be better about managing my fears as a person who will be continuing to live with this disease.

~ Kate

You must have incredible inner strength to withstand those terrifying periods of waiting to hear what is going on inside your body. How do you manage it all and stay standing?

It sounds like your music has gained new meaning since your diagnosis. My violin is my proxy voice. I have a very soft real voice and have trouble singing or talking above a normal volume. In fact, whenever I have a nightmare, I am usually mute, which sometimes enters the plot in some way. So, I am in awe of people with great singing voices.

~ Alyse

I got some difficult news in the last week that has made it impossible for me to concentrate on anything. I just had a PET scan, and it turns out that my cancer is indeed growing, though it has not spread to any other organs.

The good news is that I have found a clinical trial that begins in February. The trial itself will be in Davis, so it looks like I will be going elsewhere for care for a while, but parp inhibitors are the best bet for someone with a BRCA1 mutation. I am grateful for more time, and I know I have been incredibly lucky again as I know people that have been waitlisted for trials.

~ Kate

The difficult news that you received sounds completely overwhelming to deal with on so many different emotional dimensions. I am grateful that you had a wonderful Christmas, and I hope there are many other days in which you somehow find relief from such a heavy burden.

I hope the trial runs smoothly for you, and, of course, that it does its job to keep your cancer from growing!

I took the MCAT at the end of January. Honestly, it was kind of nice to focus on a big project like that because it forced me to look closely at my health and stress levels, which I generally ignore.

~ Alyse

First off, let me apologize for this letter being so late. I think a lot of it has to do with the fact that I am simply in denial about how shitty these cancer treatments make me feel and the desire I have to write you when I am free of drugs or at least not in some altered state based on something I am taking.

Congratulations on finishing the MCAT! I know that is a lot of studying and a huge deal. Way to go!

I got in the clinical trial! The trial consists of chemo, Carboplatin, every three weeks and ABT-888 twice daily. The good news is that the trial appears to be working. When I entered the trial I had a palpable tumor in the sub-clavicle region on my left side. When I went in for my second round of chemo, my oncologist could not feel it anymore. I have to admit that the first time I went through my chemo treatment I had real concerns about quality of life. But things are getting better; the treatment seems to be working and something had to be done to knock back the cancer. It is just scary being a stage IV and knowing that everything you are doing now is to prolong your life, and sometimes it is a crapshoot.

I am currently living with my folks. I was living with my boyfriend, but the relationship came to a screeching halt, largely because the cancer was too much for him, and I moved in with my parents. Dating when you have cancer is kind of weird to say the least. When do you tell someone? Not to mention that cancer is something of a buzz kill when you are trying to meet someone new.

Thanks for being my pen pal, Alyse.

~ Kate

I hope that your most recent scan brought good news. What a terrible waiting game it must be for these kinds of results.

I think you are nothing less than heroic for enduring what sounds like an unglamorous and constant struggle while doing things in life that are challenging enough without having cancer. I hope that you try to continue dating. It sounds like a difficult and strange experience to try to reconcile being young and having cancer.

I hope that the next few months bring you equilibrium in your current treatment.

~ Alyse

Chapter 3

I Wish I Had The Answers

Polina & Luz

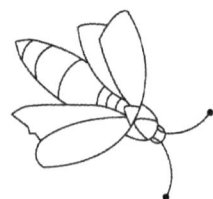

I am taking a year off between university and medical school to work as a Breast Care Center intern. I also help coordinate a drug trial called I-SPY 2. My family is from Russia, but I was born and raised in Toronto, Canada. I am 21.

In the past three months I have: finally gotten over my fear of the Operating Room, met a bunch of incredible women and men. . . but mostly women, cycled between feelings of failure and strongly held belief that I don't want to be a doctor followed by feelings of incredible commitment to medicine and to making a difference.

I am curious; what makes a good doctor? I am sure you have interacted with lots of members of the medical profession, both good and bad. Which qualities stand out?

~ Polina

I am from Spain, though I have been in the US since 1996. This makes us both European American.

I double majored in Physics and Math and then went on to do a Masters in Math. I started a PhD in Math as well, but got married and never went back to the PhD. I was working as an editor of standardized math tests, and I was so bored that I decided to go back to school and study law. Now I work in legal aid, helping victims of domestic violence with their restraining orders, family law matters and a few immigration issues. In all honesty, I did not realize how taxing this work was going to be as I am continuously surrounded by people going through one of the worst periods of their lives. At this point I have to take time off to reevaluate.

What makes a good doctor? I can tell you that my favorite doctors have been great scientists, first and foremost. Accurate and precise. If I need hand-holding I will go to family, friends, or whatever, but from my doctor I expect adequate medical information, timely diagnostic tests, appropriate treatment options. Also, I expect a doctor to realize that I am able to understand what a bell curve is, and regression analysis, and general statistical terms and that they can talk to me at a certain level.

Paternalism and condescension from a doctor who is treating you for a deadly disease is unbearable, truly adding insult to injury. Last, but not least, a modicum of empathy is nice, but very secondary to the most elemental respect due to any other human being even though you are disrobed, mutilated or about to be mutilated, cooked or about to be cooked, and generally robbed of the most basic options that people have.

~ Luz

It is hard to imagine a job where you are helping people who need it but also dealing with overwhelmingly difficult and sad situations. Do you think that your experience with cancer allowed you to relate to these women? The women that I have met so far in the breast cancer clinic are more inspiring than depressing. They are so optimistic, so insistent on being kind even though they deserve more than anyone to be grouchy, and so resilient to pain and suffering. Or is that just the face that I see in the clinic?

Your thoughts on what makes a good doctor were really interesting. I am sure you are better equipped to get scientific knowledge than most patients, but I expect that most doctors don't take the time to figure that out.

~ Polina

Having my son is the most singular event in my life, and the best. Producing another human being is truly remarkable. And then being told, while he is an infant, that you are sick like you never imagined and will not be able to take care of him for years to come; that you cannot run after him in the park while on chemo because you may have a cardiac event; that if you want to freeze eggs to preserve the possibility of giving him a sibling it would be against medical advice, as it would delay the commencement of your treatment, which would severely further compromise your chances of survival; that the radiation treatment may cause cancer; oh, and that is if you last long enough, there is a significant risk that as a side effect of the chemotherapy you will develop leukemia. Do you have any questions? I burst into laughter and asked the very serious team why they didn't just shoot me.

~ Luz

I am so sorry that you had to come up with the strength to accept those decrees that the doctor gave you. I am so sorry that you now have to live in the day to day while also thinking about such stark realities. I am sorry that it all came after you were already transitioning to a new country and to having a child.

One thing I have enjoyed this year while working and not being in school is being able to discover my intellectual passions in the absence of any evaluation, whether it is grades or other people's opinions. It has been fun to see that I actually spend time reading or thinking about what could I do "for fun?" I hope that confession doesn't make me seem like a terribly Type A pre-med, or lifeless. I am quite responsible, and often that means having trouble distinguishing between what I want to do and what I have to do.

Tell me about your son, Luz.

~ Polina

Tomas is now seven. Just thinking about him brings a smile to my face. He is a happy dude and a ham. He is always in a good mood. He prances and skips around rather than walking. He hums and sings to himself, he plays with Legos. When he was four years old, I used to listen to a Led Zeppelin CD in the car when I drove him to preschool, and he loved the CD, in particular the immigrant song. About the cancer and Tomas, we don't really tell him too many specifics. He is very aware that I am, generally speaking, kind of delicate and in relatively poor health, but that is the extent of that. I live with Damocles' sword hanging over my head; my husband lives with it as well. But Tomas does not. I shaved my head in front of him so that he wouldn't freak out when I became bald. He has never asked, "So, do you have cancer?"

If he did, we would answer yes.

Personally, nothing positive has come out of my cancer. I am not a better person. I am not more enlightened, I am not wiser, I don't have less time but enjoy it more. No, I just have a shorter expected life span, tons of medical bills, tons of side effects, and tons of limitations. The one thing that has helped me to get through the worst parts was reading about Eastern philosophy. For me, essentially, they adopt a universal and accepting view of the self and the world, allowing you to detach from yourself while attaching yourself to the rest of the universe in a way that brings peace.

~ Luz

Living every day with a dagger over your head. That is such a sad, difficult thing to face. I am so sorry. Having cancer doesn't mean that you don't also have the normal, unrelated struggles to deal with as well: raising a child, finding a job, cooking dinner.

One of the things I have been grappling most with is the boundaries between a doctor and patient. There are several patients that I care deeply about who have high risk disease and aren't responding to chemotherapy. How do I protect myself from taking everyone's struggles on?

Should I accept the fact that my choosing to be a doctor with empathy and human emotion means that I am implicitly taking on that emotional struggle as well? And another issue I have been grappling with: is there a good way to die? How do you face death without losing hope? Have you and your husband talked about death at all?

Thank you so much for taking the time to read my words. Thank you for entrusting me with your emotions even though I couldn't ever really understand what you are going through. Thank you for treating me as an equal and with respect for my experience, even though we are coming from such different places.

~ Polina

Has it occurred to you that it is you and the people like you, who have taken a selfless interest in the cancer patient community and are bridging the gap and helping us to not feel like lepers in our own towns, in our own lives?

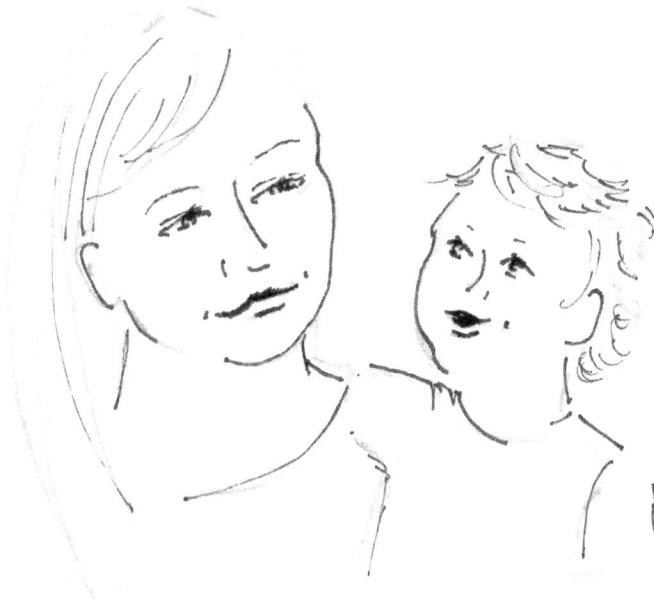

The fact that we live in a community that lives with its back towards death, denying it, rather than integrating it in the narrative of life, makes it virtually impossible for a patient with a terminal disease, or a gravely ill patient, to talk just about anything that goes through his or her mind. If you choose to be a doctor who treats patients, this means you will be seeing sick patients every day, Polina. If you are empathetic, empathize. If you are aware of what's eating you as a doctor, then you can also take care of yourself and be well-balanced.

My dearest grandmother died between our letters. Fortunately, I had enough time to go to Spain, give her a bunch of hugs and kisses and hang out with her and kind of see her off, and then she died. I loved her immensely.

My husband, Erik, and I have talked a lot about death. I have to make a will and set up a trust for my son, but the truth is that I have been dragging my feet (but then, I drag my feet with all things administrative!). Erik is five years younger than me, so I suppose that he will remarry after I die, which is kind of nice for my son's sake.

~ Luz

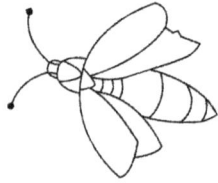

Becca & Kathy

Hiking is definitely one of my favorite activities. You, too, right? I heard that you hiked the Appalachian trail. What was that like?

I am originally from Massachusetts and lived there my whole life, so moving out to California has been an adventure in itself. It seems like every day I discover something new and amazing in this city, like eight varieties of peaches and nectarines with names like "spice zee"?

I am working at the UCSF Breast Care Center doing a cost effective analysis of two different types of radiation treatments after breast cancer surgery. Another part of my job is called "Decision Services." We call patients who are coming for their first visit at the Breast Care Center and offer to send them videos, help them prepare a list of questions for their doctor's appointment, attend the first visit with them and take notes and make an audio recording and send them a typed summary. I am doing all this while thinking about medical school.

~ Becca

I hiked the Appalachian Trail with my mom who was 62 at the time. We hiked over 2000 miles between April and October, 2006. All the hikers came to know us as the mother and daughter team who survived breast cancer. We were north bounders. We began in Georgia as soon as the snow melted and finished up in Maine before it got too cold. Once we made up our minds and figured out how to cover our bills while we were away, we asked our jobs for leaves of absences and hit the trail. If it wasn't for the "pause" breast cancer introduced into both of our lives, we wouldn't have pushed the envelope and lived that dream. My trail name was Lefty. As you probably guessed, I had breast cancer in the left breast. My mom's trail name was Righty.

I was diagnosed with breast cancer at age 31. I found the lump myself. After surgery, chemo and radiation the waiting game began. I was fortunate. I feel pretty confident nine years out that we got it all. I have had a number of close friends, also young adults, who were not so lucky and have since died from their cancers.

Why I survived and they didn't, I will never know. What I do know is that I have learned a tremendous amount about living and dying from these friends who allowed me to accompany them along their final years, months, days and hours. They are the reason I decided to shift careers and now work in end-of-life care.

~ Kathy

Do you keep in touch with any of the thru hikers you met on the trail? I have gone on a few trail-building trips and led a couple of outdoor orientation trips for college freshmen and after just a week in the woods together, we are as close as if we've known each other for years. It is something about being a bit out of our comfort zone, with no work or technology distractions and plenty of time to tell stories, play games and make amazing back-country meals together that builds lasting friendships.

Are there any frustrations that you have had during or after treatments? What do you think of sending song lyrics back and forth?

~ Becca

A song by Melissa Etheridge comes to mind. I had been a fan of hers for over ten years before she got breast cancer and wrote this amazing song, "I Run for Life."

I run for hope.
I run to feel.
I run for the truth for all that is real.
I run for your mother, your sister, your daughter, your wife.
I run for you and me my friend. I run for life.

This was the theme song for me during my hike in 2006, Becca. I listen to it every day and each time it moves me as if I was listening to it for the very first time.

When I felt a lump in my breast, I knew something was wrong. After giving me a breast exam, my doctor's exact words were, "You don't have anything to worry about, Kathy.

You are too young for this to be cancer. And, it is too large. It is probably a bunch of cysts together." When I insisted on being very worried, she said I could come back in a month. All I gleaned from our conversation was that radiology would be the next step. Since I was working in the financial district at the time, I goggled radiology offices within walking distance, walked into one during my lunch break and asked if I could be seen by a doctor. They performed the imaging that same day. Within a day or two I was diagnosed with grade three ductal carcinoma and scheduled for surgery. Chemo and radiation followed. A couple of weeks after my diagnosis, I received a phone call from my doctor. She apologized profusely, and said she was incredibly surprised by the cancer outcome.

~ Kathy

My song for this letter is, "Eye of the Tiger." This song has popped up at opportune times: road races, the teaching fellows in my organic chemistry class played it for everyone before our final exam, and most recently, I listened to it before taking my MCAT.

It is the eye of the tiger, it is the thrill of the fight,
Risin' up to the challenge of our rival
And the last known survivor.
Stalks his prey in the night –
And he is watching us all with the Eye of the Tiger.

~ Becca

It is amazing how full, even to the point of overwhelm, life can get sometimes, isn't it? I feel like the number one priority in my life is to continue slowing down, getting quieter and doing less, Becca. I recently realized that I am a "recovering extrovert". I say that with a smile on my face. One year ago today I committed to a daily morning meditation practice. On my one-year anniversary I decided to make another commitment to myself. I committed to living this next year as if it were my last. I first stumbled across Stephen Levine's book, "A Year To Live", in 2003 during my breast cancer treatments. This is my year! MY year to live.

~ Kathy

Yesterday I was feeling pretty stressed and couldn't shake the tension from my body. I biked down to Ocean Beach to watch the sunset. It was chilly and windy, but I had a warm jacket on so the breeze on my face felt good. I walked up and down the beach just letting my senses absorb my surroundings: the shouts of children, the smell of the bonfires, the rippling of kites struggling to take off from the sand. I stayed for awhile after sunset, thinking about, how for me, this was my meditation. Why did I always wait until I was stressed to bike down to the beach? This is my commitment to myself from now on. Maybe not every day, but I will start with once a week.

Thank you, Kathy, for your warmth and reflection in everything you have shared in the letters.

~ Becca

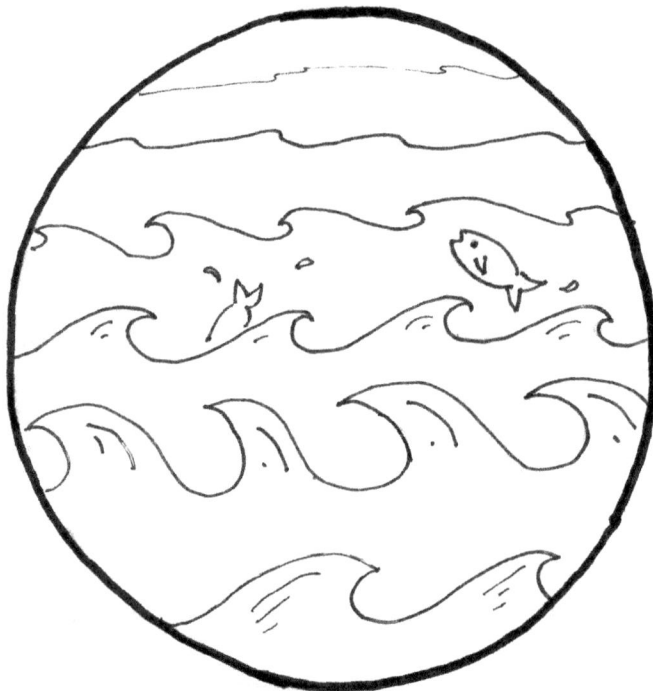

Evie &Todd

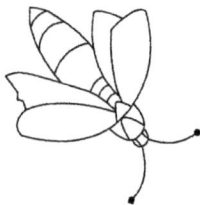

I am finding my anxiety about writing this first line paralyzing, so here it goes unedited: I am 22, a premedical intern. It was thus the cosmos aligned, and we were chosen to embark upon this journey together!

I am going to try a not so conventional approach to describing myself. Today I woke up at 7:00 am. I checked my work email, popped open Microsoft excel and did a little number crunching and color-coding while gobbling up a bowl of Cheerios in my favorite bowl – the blue ceramic one. I wound up at work at 9:00 am, a bit late, but in time to call a patient to help her develop a list of questions before her appointment with an oncologist. Later I helped one of my bosses polish up a proposal we are writing to fund a power yoga intervention for breast cancer patients. Every time I have done yoga in the past, I have been unable to contain my laughter at how absurdly impossible some of the poses seem to me. Today is day one of me respecting the process. No more giggles.

~ Evie

I, too, am finding my own anxiety about writing my first letter, so know you are not alone. When it comes to writing, it is something that I don't especially look forward to. I don't think I have ever enjoyed the process. I get too overly concerned with how my words come out, and find myself spending hours upon hours trying to get my thoughts on paper. So, like you, I am just going to write as if I am talking to you.

I am 45 years old, born in Texas, lived there until I was six and my parents got divorced, and I was whisked away to Carson City, Nevada. My family life has not been ideal. I was more the mama's boy, while my older brother was a daddy's boy. At the age of 18 I quickly departed and moved to Reno to go to college. I had no idea what I wanted to do with my life.

I finally accepted my "gayness" when I was about 22 years old. I came out, and I have never regretted being gay. I actually embrace the life and would want no other sexuality. I have now been teaching for 20+ years, 15 years now at an incredible private school, basically the Garden of Eden when it comes to education.

In August of 2002 I was diagnosed as being HIV positive. I don't blame anyone other than myself for whatever careless mistakes I made in the past. Instead I chose to embrace the disease and find a way to make something of it. So I currently teach a 11th and 12th grade Human Anatomy class where I diagnose each student with a chronic condition, and they have to live with it for three months, learning as much as they can.

I realize that I am getting older. I am more aware of how things aren't working like they used to. I start to think about what my life is NOW going to be like, as I get older. What does it all mean? I try to be positive, but then I start to fret and wonder: can I make the mortgage? Will I be alone? What will I do when Mila, my dog, passes?

~ Todd

Todd, your frankness about all the challenges you have faced and how you handled them, as well as your constant determination to do better at every point in your life, kept me reading and re-reading your letter. I have been pretty much on a track my whole life, and it is really inspiring to see all that can come by having the strength it takes to make real changes. For now, I feel like I really do want to be on my current path, but it is always good to check in with myself.

Sometimes I feel a little locked in with my goal of becoming a doctor. I see myself as going through a long training period that spans my 20s and then plops me in one place for the rest of forever, in all likelihood. I won't have those spontaneous adventures that so many other people seem to have in their 20s and 30s, enjoying the beautiful serendipity of life, because I will be in one place for four years, another for three to six years and then possibly another. I don't want medicine to be my whole life. At the same time, I know I am fascinated by the mystery of chemicals in the body, the complex mechanics of a skeleton, muscles, joints and nerves all tangled together. The idea of helping someone regain their ability to live their life how they want to truly empowers me.

I don't know very much about what it means to be HIV positive. What has it been like for you, if it is okay to ask?

~ Evie

You are right where you are supposed to be, dealing with this thing called LIFE the best way you know how. Your life parallels mine in so many ways. Let me put it in terms of biology. Life is like a cell membrane, a fluid mosaic model, never static, ever changing! Realize all the concerns you have will take care of themselves; just enjoy the adventure while you can. You just never know how long your adventure will last.

I am also trying to go with what I feel, sense, believe to be right. For some reason I feel that what you are doing regarding your career choice is right on track. What you wrote was so genuine and passionate. I knew from that point that if you can just enjoy the experience, the spontaneity and adventure will all come.

Living with HIV. . . well, it has been nine years. In a nut shell: the sero-converting phase was gruesome. It was a week of misery. The diagnosis, of course, was shocking, like any diagnosis I am sure. Lots of emotions: grief, anger, defenseless, hopelessness, acceptance and REBIRTH. Now it is fairly easy to control. One pill in the morning, two pills at night. Blood work every three months. It is about just being aware that I have this with me for life.

~ Todd

> I really want to make these letters count, Todd, but the pressure is paralyzing.
>
> ~ Evie

Let go of any pressure to make your letters count. Whatever comes from our exchanges is what we were meant to have. Whatever we get from this experience will serve its purpose now and throughout our lives.

I have noticed as I have gotten older my thoughts do often turn to life purpose, meaning and value. What I guess I am trying to get at is that I think you know that life can be short, difficult, challenging, unfair, and so many other words, but, Evie, if anything comes from our interactions, just always look at the bigger picture. All I guess I am saying is that I realize now I am one of those older people I used to talk about in high school or in my 20s, "Oh, when I get that old, or when I am that age, I hope I don't. . ."

But now in my 40s I realize how fortunate we all are to have a chance to live an existence here on Earth.

~ Todd

My last letter. This day has really come too soon. We are just getting somewhere.

Working with patients every day has helped me to step outside of myself. So many women have done absolutely nothing wrong and yet have breast cancer; they have to endure hard-hitting toxic chemotherapy, have their breasts removed, suffer from hair loss, immune system problems, gastrointestinal, cognitive, psychological and sexual problems and not just during treatment but sometimes forever onward. What compounds the suffering of so many is that they are caught completely by surprise, amplifying the injustice. A majority of cases spring up in women without any family history, and many cases seem to happen in people who had little reason at all to think they were high risk.

It is not just breast cancer patients who have opened my eyes, though. I have come to see how common it is for people to have some handicap in their quality of life. They may be thriving overall, but often struggle with something. That is just life.

Todd, it has been a real joy and powerful experience writing with you. And, with that I will close with your words: how fortunate we all are to live an existence here on earth. I couldn't agree more! From one lucky human being to another, thank you.

~ Evie

Ah, the final letter. Yes, I agree, we were finally getting somewhere. But, unfortunately, I need to keep this letter short, as I have to teach my class in 30 minutes and I am not as prepared as I should be. I have fallen victim to procrastinating lately. I know I preach to my students, but I fail to put into action what I tell them.

I want to convey how appreciative I am for your listening to me ramble on in my letters, and how important and meaningful your sharing your stories has meant to me. To good friends and lives filled with happiness. Stay strong. Be sure to smile. Peace and love.

~ Todd

Ben & Evalyn

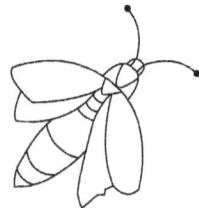

My name is Ben, and I am a second-year medical student. That is how I have started hundreds of emails over the years to people that I don't know. I am interested in many things, but I have pursued few areas to any substantial depth. One thing I can say with confidence is that I love to laugh and to make people laugh.

Of course, we have been put in touch because you are coping with cancer. Is that something that I should think about as I try to piece together a concept of who Evalyn is?

~ Ben

This year has been and will continue to be centered on making people laugh, because, in the final analysis, if we can't laugh at even those things that make us weep, how is survival possible?

My cancer diagnosed, operated on and cured in the space of 100 days of this past summer, gave me plenty of reason to mourn and tremble in the corner of my bedroom – and I did plenty of both. Finally, not only was I able to smile at the final path report that gave me an "all clear," I was also able to find a rueful smile or two during the entire terrifying process mainly because of the treatment I received at the hands of medical professionals like you.

To respond to your questions about whether or not I would like to talk about my cancer, let me say this about that: let's discuss it all. In fact, I need to, and I would love to hear your experiences with patients. What does it feel like to work with the failing human body as your life's work?

~ Evalyn

I am glad that you had such positive experiences in the hospital. In reality, however, doctors and nurses are human and as such, respond best to those patients who are pleasant, respectful and understanding.

As a second-year medical student, most of my time is spent in a classroom-learning environment. I do interact with patients, but those interactions are limited. As I transition to full time clinical training where I see patients every day, your questions about doctor/patient relationships are very relevant for me since I have not yet formed or refined my approach.

I have never thought about medicine in the terms of working with the failing human body, even though I understand that it is a fitting description. I think I am working with the human body, an incredibly complex entity. I am so passionate about the human aspect of medicine, working together with people on issues that are personal and important for them.

Not all doctors deal with death on a regular basis. I deal with thoughts about my own death the way that most people, especially young people, do, by assuming that it is too far off to worry about right now. Working on that assumption, I am much more concerned right now with my parent's death than my own. For them, as well as myself, I can only wish that when death comes we can look back with satisfaction on the life we have lived.

~ Ben

When I first got the diagnosis with the large fibroid, before finding out it had a touch of cancer in it, I named her FIONA THE FABULOUS FIBROID. However, after the diagnosis, I lost my sense of humor a bit.

As you transition from classroom learning about medicine to full time clinical training, give serious thought to your approach. I am telling you right now to start thinking of your patients as people first, patients second. You are, after all, dealing with people who are terrified of what is happening to them.

Deciding now that you want to either dive into their humanity full throttle or simply exist on the level where medicine is medicine may decide what kind of doctor you will be.

We all die, young and old. No one gets out of life alive. It is huge and true, so along with your studies on the body as a machine, how to fix it, make it work better, I wonder if matters of the spirit enter into your training at all? Personally, my Buddhism and daily deep meditation saved me during my cancer scare last summer. In Buddhism, there is no real belief that death is a final thing, but rather merely one of the changes all forms of energy undergo throughout the universe. I now know, after having cancer in my body, that death is a very real thing, and that we are all fragile as can be. I think of death every day, meditate on it every morning.

I also have fears I didn't have before. Maybe I did have them, but they were only lying in wait for something to wake them up – fear of something bad happening.

But you know what? BAD THINGS DO HAPPEN, every hour of the day and night to many, many people and one day, bad things will happen to all of us. It is part of life. Onward I plod, reveling in the man who loves me, the friends I love, the cookies I must bake and the presents I must wrap, and somehow, we all get through.

~ Evalyn

In a way, Evalyn, medical education is not set up to teach medical students to think of patients as people. Patients are largely theoretical entities. We learn all about disease after disease and we talk about it; patients are more of an abstract concept. Matters of the spirit do not enter into our training much if at all. Neither are spirituality or religion an important part of my life. I am very interested in how people's faith can help them through difficult medical circumstances.

~ Ben

Well, there is not much left to say, except there is always so much to say about the subjects of illness, cancer, death, life and living.

I have been cancer-free now for over six months and have gone back to my normal life almost as if nothing ever happened to make me realize how short life really is. As I get closer and closer to re-engaging with the memories, my feelings get more and more tender, Ben.

Cancer robs us of our most valuable possessions. It is a thief we cannot bring to justice. Ever. Death always wins in court. Illness, well, we can put it off for a while, but ultimately, it wins too. I wish I had answers. But I do not.

One thing I am positive about: meeting you and my other pen pals. This has been one fabulous way to spend some of the time I have on this earth. People matter more to me now than they ever did before. And each taste of food is more delicious.

Each experience, sad or happy, pulsates more with the flavors of living than ever before.

~ Evalyn

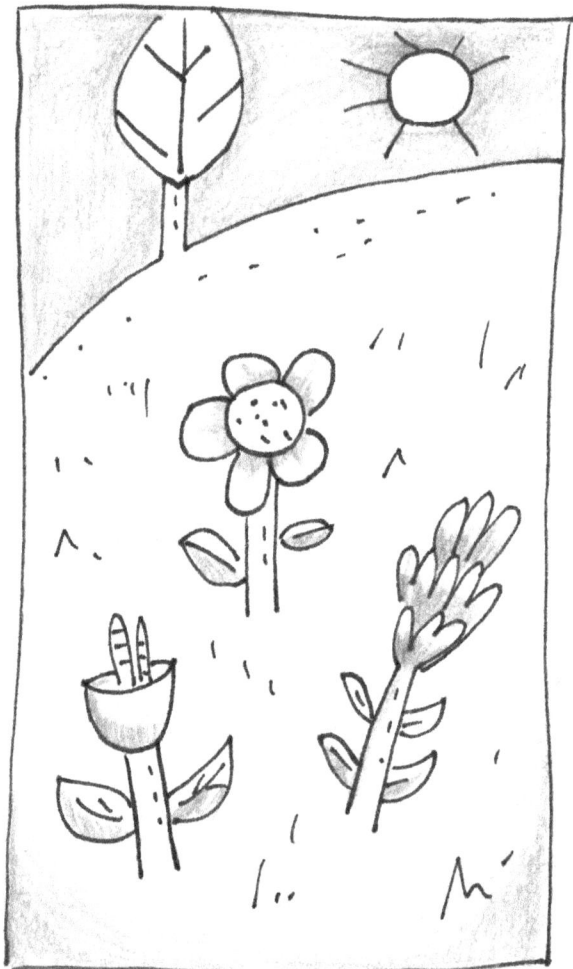

Sam & Evalyn

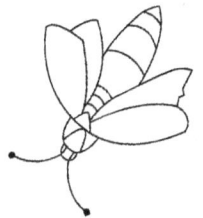

I am a fourth-year medical student at UCSF. I would like to be an oncologist. Some of my most moving experiences in school so far have been with cancer patients. I grew up in the Bay Area and went to Harvard for college. I came running back to San Francisco as fast as I could after graduating, mostly because of the cold winters in Boston.

I heard you were nominated for a Tony Award. How wonderful it must be to perform at such a high level. I love to sing, and performing is a big part of my life. In fact, I played Tony in "West Side Story" in college. It is what keeps me sane when I am working too hard.

~ Sam

Harvard and Tony in *West Side Story* AND you want to use your medical training to be an oncologist! You sound absolutely perfect to me!

My brush with uterine cancer has a happy ending, at least for now. If there is one thing I have learned from this terrifying experience, it is that anything can happen to any of us at any time, so I treat all of life now with a new sensitivity, an awareness made sharper by every moment of the fear I felt throughout those days. It was like being on another planet, or like in the hill caves of a country far, far away. I am changed as a result of it, changed utterly.

Yes, I was a Tony nominee in 1985 for a show called *Quilters* on Broadway. But now I have moved to San Francisco with my darling husband, and devote my time to writing. I am writing a book and a monthly column for the Marina Times. I adore theater, have adored it all my life, and now it feels good to be in the audience, not on the stage. Why did you choose medicine over being an actor?

~ Evalyn

Wow, you were nominated the year I was born! 1985! I think perhaps it is difficult for someone like me, who has never experienced cancer, to understand what a "brush" with cancer is truly like. My family has experienced cancer, but each time it was relatively easy to treat. It wasn't until this past year when I helped care for cancer patients as part of the medical team that I realized the true impact this disease can have on patients and their families. I had a feeling I wanted to be an oncologist even before I saw my first patient with cancer, but now I am fairly certain of it.

I learned to sing as a child by listening to pop singers on the radio. I stopped singing after I hit puberty because my awkward teenage voice was cracking all the time. I didn't get the nerve to sing again until the end of high school. I joined the beginner level chorus where the teacher pulled me aside and asked if he could give me private lessons. One day, I got up in front of the whole school and sang Beauty and the Beast. It was such a cool moment for me. I was met with a standing ovation. From that moment, I have been singing nonstop. Let's put together a list of our favorite songs.

Coming out of college, I debated pursuing music instead of medicine. In the end, I decided that pursuing medicine while keeping music as a hobby would be more feasible than the other way around. I still have dreams of being a world famous pop star, but that life is not for me.

I have questions for you about your experience with cancer. Of course, if anything makes you uncomfortable, please feel free to not answer them. How did you first realize something was wrong? How did the doctor break the news to you? I think one of the hardest things for me as an oncologist will be to deliver bad news to a patient. It is not often that I have the opportunity to ask these questions of someone who has experienced this disease.

As we've been putting together a list of our favorite songs, I'd like to add the song "Somewhere" to our list. This song truly speaks to me. I know what it feels like to be out of place, not feeling like I belong. We should try to get together and sing.

~ Sam

If there is one thing I have learned from this, it is that there is no scale for suffering. When one suffers, one suffers! Thoughts of death are with me every single day in a way that they have never been before. And this is me, now, with no cancer! IT HAS OPENED MY EYES! And I am the wiser for it. Even the air tastes better to me. That, of course, may be a function of the simple fact that I now live in the glorious San Francisco, not obnoxious New York City. I am vigilant for what may come next because, ultimately, something will come next.

How did I find out I had cancer, you ask? The doctor waited until after the weekend, even though she knew I had cancer late the previous Friday afternoon. Looking back on it, I am glad she waited. Her phone call was brief, warmly spoken and to the point. She expressed her surprise that they found something; it had all looked clean to her. But I remember thinking, "Now I am a statistic, and I am going to die sooner rather than later." I was in her office 20 minutes later filling out paperwork.

I did withdraw after my diagnosis, somewhat, and I also chose carefully the people I told. I wanted no "puppy eyes" filled with pity. I just wanted to get through it and try not to die from fear. I sat and meditated, and it saved my life.

I really didn't go into remission as much as it was totally cut out of me. It had not spread beyond the uterus. But I was so relieved; it took me several days to trust that when the phone rang, it wasn't the oncologist's office calling me to say they had made a mistake – and that I was filled with the dreaded, nasty, vile, cruel, evil, senseless, goddamned disease. And for now I had beaten it. I had, for now, overcome it.

Grateful does not describe it. Even the air began to sparkle. I was immediately starving for food; I wanted to drink an entire bottle of Scotch. I let the few people I had told know the good news. People wept; so did I.

~ Evalyn

Your vivid descriptions are so touching. It is so great to meet you. My life is busy. I have a habit of working too hard, and this year I am in a research laboratory studying new therapies for leukemia. Each day is an intellectual challenge and a steep learning curve. It is sometimes difficult to keep in mind the impact my work could one day have on people with cancer, especially when I am particularly stressed or sleep deprived.

I am lucky I live close to my family. My parents are both doctors and my younger brother wants to become a doctor also.

~ Sam

Whew, two parents who are doctors! No pressure there, right? Yikes!

~ Evalyn

My parents actually tried to persuade me to pursue something other than medicine for the longest time. I really appreciated that, because I really felt able to make my own decision. I think a love for medicine just runs in my veins. I am grateful for many things, especially for being able to live my life openly. No matter what life brings us, there are so many things to be grateful for, like finally meeting you!

~ Sam

Growing up means accepting death as a part of life. It means accepting that there are fine doctors and nurses who dedicate their lives to making our lives easier, less painful and more possible. Time is ours to spend. And we really should learn to spend it well.

Life is the only thing we know, isn't it? None of us knows what awaits us after it. We only know if we have good lives worth living, and I have one, that if we lose this life, we lose being with the people we love, we lose sharing more of life's adventures with those who make life the wonderful thing it is.

~ Evalyn

Chapter 4
This Is What The Living Do

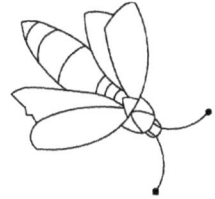

Brandon P. & Margo

My mother once told me I shouldn't talk with strangers, but she never mentioned letter writing. So, I suppose this is okay. I am 22 years old and I am working on figuring out what that means. I moved to San Francisco this past summer after graduating college in Boston, at Harvard. Well, technically it is in Cambridge. I am working as a pre medical intern at UCSF. I am applying to medical school, which is a drain on my time, energy and savings. Having said that, if medical school applications are my biggest worry, I must be in a good place.

After working here for only a couple of months, I already feel like I need to return to the kind of work I was doing in college and before. I have been involved in HIV/AIDS and LGBT health issues since I was 16. Working in these arenas is how I found medicine as a career and in many way it is where I found the best parts of myself. What gets you all fired up? Excited? Thrilled? Pissed off?

I collect old medical educational materials, buttons used in AIDS protests. I also collect licenses and certifications. I was SCUBA certified, I have a bartending license, could legally operate most anything that floats, just got my motorcycle license, was a Red Cross certified safe babysitter, and I am an ordained minister. It seems unlikely that I will be able to use all of these at the same time, but I do enjoy the image of bartending at an underwater motorcycle marriage chapel.

I also have to acknowledge that a big part of why we are exchanging letters is that you have cancer. What parts of the story are you willing to tell? How long have you been living with it? I would be interested in answers of any size. As a way of getting to know one another a little it, I would love to hear about some of your rituals, the things you do with regularity that bring you structure, meaning, joy and peace, whatever. For instance, I wear a bow tie to work every Wednesday. I go to Church and talk with my mother most Sundays. That sort of thing.

I have one more question I would like to ask you. I interviewed a group of men who had been involved in very early AIDS activism and I would like to ask you the same question I used to end those interviews (my favorite question): what makes you fabulous?

~ Brandon P.

You tell me your mother says do not talk to strangers? Your mother is right. However, I am not much stranger than anyone else.

I have a diagnosis of metastatic gastric/esophageal junction stage IV cancer. I share this up front by way of letting you know I don't think I have been a very good friend to my friends. I believe that the cancer and the treatment thereof has made me more selfish, sheltered, angry, distant, indifferent, and disillusioned, broken down, weak and tired. BUT, please do know that I have also experienced some of my greatest joy, contentment and loving surrender to what is to be. My self-selected little family of friends are here with me, no matter how tired I get. I just wish I could be more for them.

Why do you want to be a pen pal with a 52-year-old Jewish lesbian with glasses, a bum shoulder, waning memory and hearing, and stage IV GE Junction cancer? Sounds like a handful when I say it like that.

My mother died when I was 16 years old. I graduated high school, moved to Marin County, went to college and then went to UC Hastings College of the Law. Katy is my forever love. We were married on October 25th, 2008. My heart. She is so stubborn, and I am equally impatient, but we sure laugh a lot. I tell her that I love her more than the moon and all of the stars, even the ones not born yet. True statement.

Since my diagnosis in January 2009, I have been on so many chemicals, radiation, opiates, cannabinoids, and Ativan, that my mind often goes mushy some days. Sometimes I can't remember what I was going to say. Sometimes we play a game at home with friends, where we sit around trying to guess what I was going to say. I do talk too much, too fast AND way too loud, use a trillion verbal commas and exclamation marks in my sentences and laugh at myself a lot!

I thought I would never say these words "Please meet MY oncologist!" When I was diagnosed, my doctors took me in. My surgeon told me that I was part of his family now. And he visited me nearly every day, in ICU and the hospital, even one Sunday with his son, who was wearing a crisp little white karate outfit.

"What makes me fabulous?" I don't think I know. Additionally, that question assumes I think that I am fabulous. In part that is the process I am going through now. Jury is out on me. We'll see.

~ Margo

I was so excited to see your first letter, I texted my roommate to let her know how cool I thought this program was. She asked what you were like. I, feeling a bit foolish, had to admit that I had no idea because I hadn't yet opened your letter.

Why do I want to be your pen pal? Well, truth be told, I am not sure I fully understand what drove me to participate. I think part of it was curiosity. I see a lot of patients coming through the clinic, but I rarely have an opportunity to get to know them. On an admittedly more self-serving level, I want to be a doctor, and I intend to be the best one I can be. I hope to learn something in our letter exchange to take with me on the next steps of my journey to becoming a physician.

Thank you for your candor about your diagnosis. I have no idea what that experience must be like, to be dealing with chronic illness and feeling like you are not the friend you wish you could be. Like a lot of LGBT identified people, I consider my closest friends to be a major part of my family.

I am in the application process now, as I mentioned before. If I could be anywhere for medical school, I would either be here at UCSF or back at Harvard. I applied to a countless number of other schools, but we'll see how this process turns out.

~ Brandon P.

At this time I am having a difficult time writing. I found out that my sister, Renee, committed suicide. She was ten months younger than I. I was adopted and my brother was adopted; then my mother got pregnant with my sister. My sister suffered tremendously from mental illness since she was about 20 or so. She died on July 28th. Just like that! Boom! Felt like a big iron cannon ball was shot into my chest at point blank range.

My life's dream is to travel to Japan, China, India, Israel, Vietnam and Thailand. I am a little scared to travel, though I do, and will, but since I have such gastrointestinal challenges, it is hard to eat just anything, anywhere. For a period of my treatment I craved, of all things, steamed clams. I could not get enough of them. My insatiable clam hunger was only problematic when Katy and I were on the road traveling. In a way, it was something that both Katy and I could do, was tangible, identified and was in a strange way, uniting.

You asked me what I meant by the statement "I want to be a friend a friend would want to have." So many of my friends came to my aid when I got THE diagnosis. For some reason I think that people liked me more once they heard I had cancer. The world, ironically, became a friendlier place for me after my cancer diagnosis. And yes, having cancer has affected every single thing in my life, especially my relationships.

I feel similarly as you about becoming a pen pal. Like you, I love stories and facts. I believe that I am on a journey, an Odyssey of sorts. Be well, pen pal friend. I will light a candle for you and think positive thoughts regarding your application process. I know that it is much more than simply an application process to you. I wish you everything you want and need.

~ Margo

I am writing this letter from the craziness of work. Patients and staff alike running around, running late, getting impatient, hearing good news, delivering bad news. Medicine is a microcosm I am learning, both good and bad.

I am so sorry to hear about your sister. I can't imagine what it is like to lose a sibling. I hope in the months that have followed since hearing the news you have found more answers.

I really want to be able to stay at UCSF. Tough thing is, I have to get in first. It is a grueling process, and the whole thing feels like a poorly choreographed middle school dance between you and the schools. You are figuring out if you want each school while wanting each school to want you. It's as tangled and uncomfortable as it sounds; I hated middle school.

~ Brandon P.

Thank you for your kind words about my sister's passing. My sister was the biological child of my adoptive parents. There was no major distinction growing up that my brother and I were adopted, and my sister was "the real one." My parents told me of my adoption at a very young age; I was so proud to be adopted. My dad told me that I was "chosen," therefore, in my mind, I was somehow the same or better. I skipped around elementary school bragging that I was chosen, and the rest of the lot of you just happened.

I also had heard our woolly gray rabbi say that we were the chosen people, and then my Baptist friend told me that because of being chosen, we had a second chance in the rapture. So, in my mind, I had been sitting pretty.

~ Margo

Thank you, Margo, for your willingness to let me into your life, for sharing the experience of letter writing with me.

In early May I found out I was accepted at UCSF Medical School. This is a dream come true for me. It is a big moment. This is the first time I have written down these words. I am ready to start becoming a doctor.

~ Brandon P.

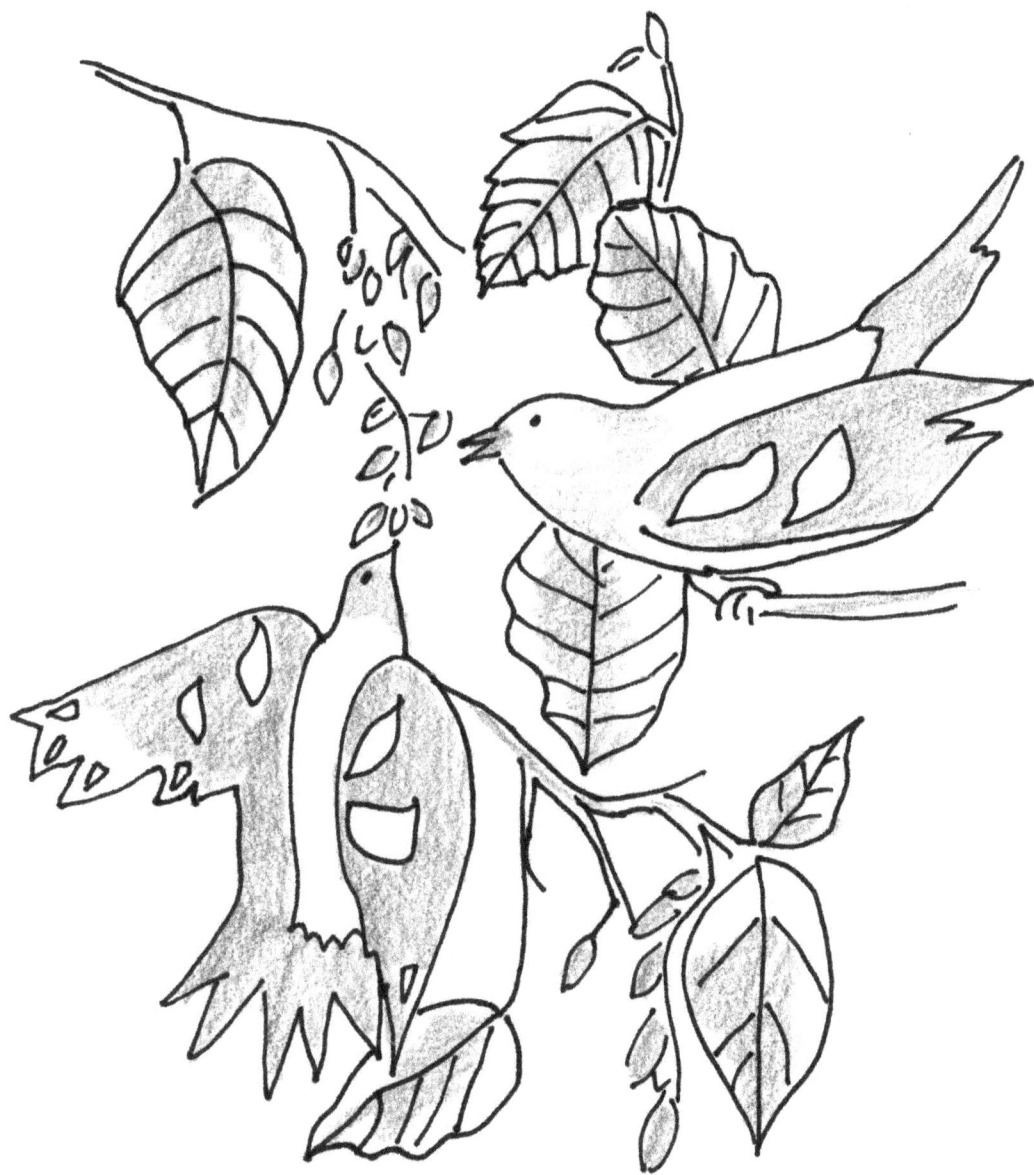

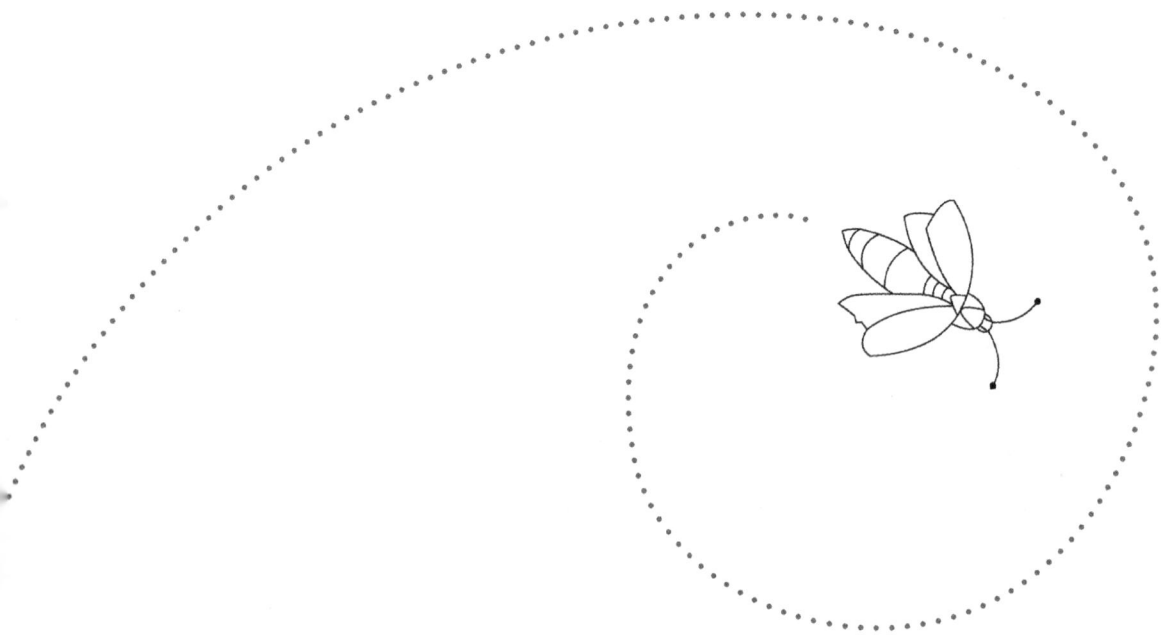

Mike & Margo

I am a medical student at UCSF, in my second year. When I found out about this program, I was surprised that patients would want to speak with medical students. If there is one thing they really drill into us, it is that we don't know anything (yet).

Omitting the boring details, I am a non-traditional student. I grew up in New England with two younger brothers and divorced parents, left for college, and basically almost partied myself to death. When I think about the person I was in my early twenties, it honestly scares me. I was selfish and made a lot of very poor and even dangerous decisions. In truth, I had wanted to be a doctor forever, but thought 2005 my grades were terrible and I had never seriously applied myself, so it seemed that that ship had sailed. But after working in finance for a few years, living out on my own and learning a little more about responsibility, my thoughts about medicine really started consuming everything.

So, I sold all my belongings, moved to San Francisco, and started over from scratch. I went back to undergraduate school here, got my EMT license, and drove an ambulance at night while attending SFSU during the day. Those three years were hard. When I finally opened the acceptance letter from UCSF I collapsed on the floor of my garage and cried. I simply could not believe that things had worked out.

I wonder every day why I got a second chance at this dream. I feel like if it wasn't something I have already done, which it is not, then it must be something I have to do in the future. I wake up with the feeling like I have to earn this all over again. I have an intense, almost manic desire to remain grateful and thankful for my life, attack challenges, and someday be good at this job.

~ Mike

It sounds as if you have had quite a journey. You must be so proud to have put that part of you in the background. I hear that you are grateful, and that seems very appropriate, but you only "owe" it to yourself to be who you were intended to be. Are you excited?

I do not know anything about you, other than what you wrote in your first letter. I don't really know a lot about anything anymore. Sometimes I do not feel "myself." But that is not exactly it; it is more like I don't "know" myself. I am, too, on a journey. This one is and has been a doozy; rich introspection. Just one of the gifts of having being diagnosed with esophageal cancer at 49 years old. So, another journey. I have had several journeys. Actually, I can't decide if I have had several journeys, over several centuries, or just one long, yet somewhat funny journey and this is my first time out of the gate.

Be forewarned, at times I may come across as direct, harsh, dark, or unyielding. But mostly, while not a positive person, I am certainly a hopeful person. And I like people, a lot. I use the word love loosely and often. I love my partner, our friends, my friends, some family and some neighbors, and our 11-year-old Jack Russell Terrier, Penny.

I did well in classes, loved school and my teachers, but couldn't wait to be free. Right before my freedom plan was to kick in, my mother got sick and died. We were in a fight. I was 16 and she was 45. She went to the hospital in the morning, on a school day, had her gall bladder removed only to pass away from a stroke late on the very same evening. My father, sister and brother moved into an alternate reality. I left home.

I have always had a funny feeling about death from an early age. My paternal grandfather died when I was about eight years old and I asked my father what it means to die, and how long does it last? He said that it lasts forever.

The long and the short: I never thought that I would ever face my own mortality and ask myself how long is forever?

I bet that you will be able to get to know your patients well. Ten minutes per patient if you are lucky. But I hope, in that brief period of time, that you treat them like family, the family that you love and care for. I have an insatiable need to forever be in the debt of those who helped me live through this disease.

~ Margo

I am very, very excited about medicine. This doesn't feel like work to me. I would probably do it for free. Second year we are starting to learn about cancer, so I am really glad to hear that you are disease free. We are assigned a preceptor, who is usually a non-UCSF physician. My preceptor is an emergency room physician and was recently handicapped, so he works from his wheelchair, and he is still, without question, the alpha dog. I was an EMT before med school, and was fairly certain I wanted to go into emergency medicine, but after working with him, I am 100% sure about that.

It is true that I always wanted to be a doctor. After college, I had been working at this hedge fund for about one and a half years, and one day I just realized this feeling would never go away, and that I would never know if I could do it unless I tried. And I couldn't live with that. So I walked over to my boss' desk and quit. Simple. It was a real awakening, catalyzed by I have no idea what.

When I went to college I played drums, drank a lot, met lots of girls and found out that all this was really just a dead end path, focused on immediate rewards, which it turns out, aren't the most rewarding, if at all. All this was probably a combination of making up for lost time, being an intense person to begin with, and just being young and not thinking at all.

~ Mike

Please feel free to ask me any question in the entire world. I likely won't be offended and certainly wouldn't be shocked, so you might as well ask me what you may wish to ask of a cancer survivor in your care. Pretend you are a doctor. I am a UCSF cancer survivor. We can be friends if we want in real life, but that is later.

To be clear, I love stories, I love the whole ball of wax, every bump, lump, wart, wrinkle, twist, happy, sad, even the tears. The more details the better, as far as I am concerned.

I think that your idea about the ER is interesting and important. You will be extremely useful to the bruised, the banged up, the dying, and their families and friends. Your education and ethic will be useful. Just by being a conscious individual with a desire to help those less fortunate than you is hugely useful.

Mike, when you become a doctor, I would love to talk to you five years into it and see how you feel.

~ Margo

Your letters just completely floor me every time. At the moment, before reading your last letter, I was stressed out about a big test we have coming up, the first step of three licensing exams we have to pass before we can treat patients on our own. It determines a lot about our future, and it is really expensive and hard. We are all putting in a lot of hours and making ourselves miserable.

But now I guess I should write "miserable" in quotes, because after hearing about the things that keep ending up in front of you and blocking your path, it seems embarrassing and ridiculous to complain about sitting in a comfy little room, eating snacks. That is probably not the point of a pen pal, to compare myself to someone, but I want you to know that the things you have been telling me have really made a difference, and stirred up some really confusing but amazing thoughts in my head. I can't wait to meet you.

~ Mike

As you are likely beginning to realize, I have had a lot of struggle in my life. I am not complaining, really. I don't feel like a victim, either; in fact, if you ask me I will, without being Pollyanna about it, tell you that I am an extremely lucky person, but I have to say that I do get weary. Trying to fix, help, understand, all while remaining compassionate, and live my own life is a tall order.

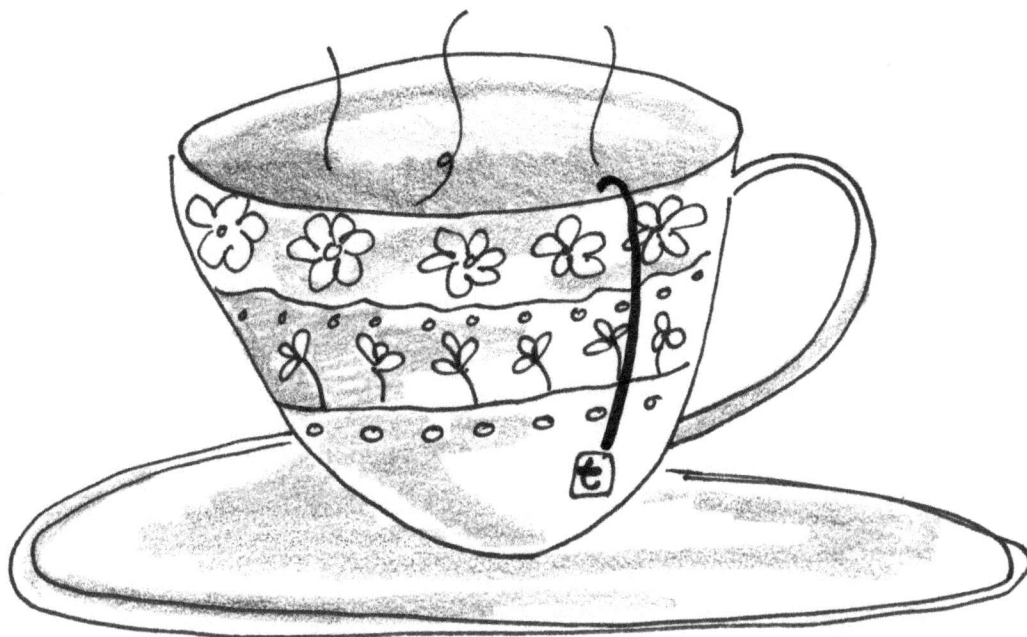

Sounds like you are on a grueling schedule. I admire that you, Mr. Pen Pal are a truly committed person. It impresses me because sometimes I think that I have flittered away good years because of my lack of commitment to an activity or goal. I can't believe that you have even a moment to write such thoughtful letters to me.

I have to have a PET/CT scan. I have put it off twice because I am tired of living with my cancer. I prefer to live for many other reasons, however. But, reality is that I need to keep up with the beast. You know the stats on metastatic esophageal cancer. While I am beating them for now, I still have a kernel of absolute terror that it will rear its bastardly head again.

Be well my new friend. Try to relax just for a minute. I will be thinking of you and your poor brain after this leg of your journey is complete. Eat well, and drink coconut water.

~ Margo

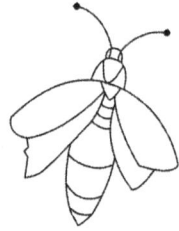

Brandon I. & Pierre

I strive to adopt a laid back approach and hope to never take any situation, or myself, too seriously. My tendency is to remember the good times and let the more difficult moments slip from memory. I am an extrovert and really enjoy the company of others.

I studied chemistry and then worked in business for a few years. I am currently a second-year medical student at UCSF. Though it is fairly early in my training, I came to school with a fairly clear sense of my ultimate career goal, which is to practice oncology. I hope to get involved with the creation of new therapeutics and am currently deciding whether it might make sense to take an extra year in medical school to learn more about the clinical process.

I am enclosing a photograph with my letter. It is from the SFO baggage claim taken in August of 2010. I did not think too much of the picture when I snapped it with my cell phone but over the past few months it has become quite sentimental for me. The photo was taken the day I used a one-way ticket and moved across the country to San Francisco, leaving my family, most of my friends, and my former career behind. It was a day of pretty significant professional transition as well since I also started medical school the next day. Though I was apprehensive then, now, this photo symbolizes a new direction and I am excited for the future.

~ Brandon I.

You are quite an interesting guy! I, for one, hope that you pursue your inkling to work in the developments of new therapeutics, since I am currently on the last FDA approved treatment protocol. Fortunately, the treatments appear to be working so the good news is that if it continues, I may be on this for the rest of my life. The bad news is that if it works I will be on it for the rest of my life. Bottom line, I can put up with practically anything to prolong my life – that is a no-brainer. But this treatment regimen has been the most difficult one that I have been through.

I was diagnosed in December 2004 with stage IV colorectal cancer. My daughter who was 16 at that time went online and reported that I would be dead in two years. I assured her that I had other plans.

In January of 2005 I began chemo treatments and in June had my first of three liver surgeries, followed by more chemo. Following all this, I became very anxious and worried about the minutest things, which was totally out of character for me. It was as if someone else was inhabiting my body. I wanted the old me to return. I pulled out of this blue period a few months later.

I will tell you that I was born to French parents in a small town in Louisiana on the Mississippi River between New Orleans and Baton Rouge. I just came back from a week of golf, and I plan on going on a two week trip to Argentina and may go to Louisiana in January for a combination fishing trip and BCS championship game in the Superdome. But I don't want to get ahead of myself.

~ Pierre

Perhaps you have been told this already, but it is significantly easier and infinitely more meaningful to understand diseases when you have a person to remember and not just a list of symptoms.

I was moved by your optimism throughout this ordeal and wonder what skills you employ to remain upbeat? I like to think that after numerous surgeries and recurrences I would retain this approach, but I guess it is hard to predict until it is a reality.

I am entering a pretty intense phase of medical school. We take our first Medical Board licensure exam, and it is a pretty daunting amount of material. Many of the older students and doctors joke that you actually know the most medicine at any point in your career the morning of the exam and the least amount right afterwards. It seems it is a right-of- passage.

~ Brandon I.

My holiday in Argentina was outstanding. It did me a lot of good. I went from barely being able to keep my eyes open to becoming energized for the remainder of the trip. I am flying to New Orleans to the BCS championship to watch the game with my brother in the comfort of his den. I plan to party in the French Quarter and enjoy some great Cajun and creole cuisine while I am in the city.

I am blessed with an innate ability to cope with the prognosis and treatment of my disease. I have an inner strength to see myself through difficult times. I don't know how to pass it on to others because I don't consciously do anything to manifest it in myself. I hope that you won't have too many tests of this power during your lifetime.

I am at a point in my treatment where I am definitely into quality of life. I am not hopeful for a cure, so I am buying time. And I want to be able to enjoy whatever time I have left. That is why I now tell my oncologist that I am going to Argentina, or Africa, and I am available for treatment until early November and resume in mid-January but must stop in May so I can feel fine for my departure to Africa in June. I have also relaxed my notion of nutrition and its benefits of warding off disease progression. It is not because I am not a believer in good nutrition. It is because food is an important part of life's pleasures for me, and so I eat whatever I want. It is all about seeking balance and attaining equilibrium that translates into happiness.

~ Pierre

Remaining upbeat, Pierre, is so important, and it looks like you have that nailed. I sincerely hope the glass remains half-full.

We are in the process of ranking various hospital sites for our third-year clinical rotations. I am not sure if you have ever played fantasy sports, but the whole process is actually quite similar to a team draft. Overall, the transition from classroom to hospital is exciting! It will be great to put many of the things we learned in books and simulations to real practice. I am not naïve to the fact that it will be incredibly challenging as well, but I tend to learn most when I am stretched a bit.

~ Brandon I.

I have played Fantasy football and the draft nights are always the most fun. But the process of ranking various hospital sites doesn't sound like much fun. Seems like you need one big mother organization program to help make the right choices.

~ Pierre

Since we last sent our letters, I received my rotation schedule, took the Board Exam, and actually started my first transitional clerkship in the hospital.

I understand that this is our last formal exchange through our letters, Pierre, and I wanted to tell you how meaningful an experience this was for me. You can read 50 papers or textbooks about cancer, but that does not teach you what it means to be diagnosed with the disease. As a budding oncologist, these letters have truly opened my eyes to many facets of cancer care that I certainly hope to apply in my own practice. Thank you for your candor and for sharing your personal thoughts about your medical care and clinical course. You have offered rich lessons and have been deeply inspiring.

~ Brandon I.

The toughest thing about being a doctor has got to be losing a patient. I suppose dealing with death on a daily basis is character building provided one doesn't burn out in the process. I applaud your inner strength to face specializing in oncology. Your patients are lucky to have someone like you looking after them.

Brandon, it has been truly great for me to have the opportunity to get a little bit inside the head and heart of a medical student, especially one who is growing into an oncologist. If I have helped you in any way to become a better doctor then there could be no higher praise.

~ Pierre

Pierre died on February 14th, 2013.

Jonathan 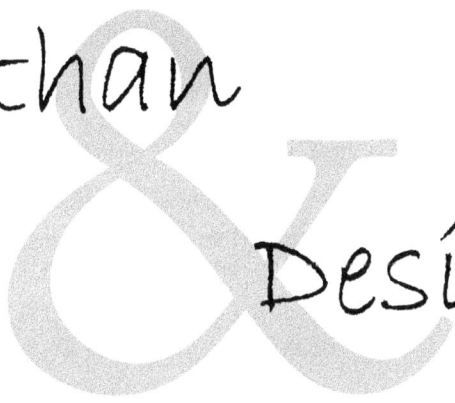 Desiree

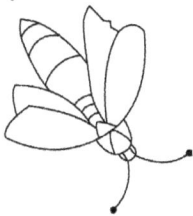

I am now one week into my Nursing Master's program, and I already feel immersed in the river of learning and responsibility, Desiree. I am struggling to remember that I can swim, and I can float, and it is not useful to be overwhelmed.

In the middle of the summer came gleeful news! I got my all-clear five-year C/T scan. I am considered cured. The first time I got a clear C/T scan five years ago, I didn't quite trust it; I didn't trust my body. I was beaten down, exhausted and still faced the looming burden dealing with my HIV status: a mountain I didn't know how to climb. And how much has happened in five years, how much has changed. This time I truly felt the news. I felt like one of the lucky ones. The ferryman of death rowed on by and let me remain on shore.

In August came my 20th high school reunion and all the old anxieties flurried around me. Nostalgically, I combed through old boxes of pieces of my teenage and childhood self. Hadn't I just been 17? Was it just a simple turning around to find myself at 38?

Time is such an elusive and slippery concept; it makes sense only on the calendar, but in the heart, mind and soul it flows around like a breeze, then slows like a gelatinous river and bends forward and arches back upon itself. The reunion itself was surprisingly joyous, and I didn't want it to end.

In the ensuing days, I yearned to do my teenage years all over again. To go back and enjoy adolescence in the ways I hadn't and be confident, to never let HIV sully my veins and depression darken my soul. I longed for innocence lost and things that I perhaps never had.

I finally was able to take my nursing boards and I am finally an RN. The Master's program has been fast, furious, exciting and challenging. Sometimes I am so overwhelmed, I just have to remember to breathe, to put one foot in front of the other, and remember to enjoy the journey.

I went to see the film 50/50 with my father. It brought back the surreal moment when the doctor told me that I had cancer, and suddenly it was as if I was looking at myself through some kind of bizarre projector, a character in a movie, someone else's life. I had the same prognosis after my cancer returned and after it had spread despite surgery to remove it. 50/50 – the toss of a coin.

I remember the difficulty of breaking the news to my mom and how I wanted to protect her. I remember the burden of everyone's expectations, the anxiety in their eyes and the sympathy I didn't always want. I remember feeling separated from life, as if it was going on all around me and I was looking in through a window suddenly relegated to the strange and distant land of the sick. I remember crying alone in my room at night, trying to muffle my sobs in an effort not to wake my parents.

I remember the fatigue and the nausea, the nausea, the never ending nausea with no relief. I remember my dad holding my hand as I went into surgery and how afraid I felt when he had to leave me at the gates. I remember the chemo going into my veins felt like poison, and I felt I couldn't take another day. I remember feeling like I couldn't take being sick anymore and sometimes how I just wanted it to end. I just wanted to hide in my room forever with my books that brought me those momentary pieces of light. The movie triggered all of these memories and more, bringing them into sharp relief, and the tears cathartically fell. After the credits rolled, I noticed that my father was literally sobbing. I had no idea how hard it had been on him. I was deeply moved.

We pass our days in flurries of stress and mundane activities. Perhaps, when survived, cancer can be a gift, a reminder that every day and every person can be a gift, every hug, every flower, every breeze, every rain drop and every moment alive here with those that we love is a moment that will never come again and one that we should savor and cherish. The trick is to retain this awareness.

~ Jonathan

I have a hard truth to face about my cancer experience. There is just no real way to make anything of it.

People say that cancer brings its gifts, an understanding of what is important in life, a deepened experience of the everyday miracles, the loveliness of just not being dead. But the truth is, I already knew how to draw on the flowers by the side of the road for their wordless wisdom. The desert taught me that. My mother taught me that. Her death taught me that. Beautiful music taught me, not in what I heard, but in what I felt physically in my body, and the spontaneous translation of that into dance. Cancer, rather than giving me these things or deepening my appreciation of them, seems to have mutilated my faith in my right to be here.

I think what cancer did more than any other experience in my life was plunge me into the quagmire that is human suffering, fill me with an enormous desire to somehow ease that suffering and leave me with no wherewithal to do that. It filled me with a crippling fear that not only do I have no way of addressing that suffering, but that I have no defense against it.

I am flirting with getting a master's in genetic counseling. I am a true geek, and you know you are a geek when you can't wait to go to the café and get a nice soy chai latte and snuggle down with your genetics text. Suddenly the wonder is not that things go wrong. The real wonder is that anything ever goes RIGHT. I had my first consultation with my new surgeon, and everything has remained stable since my last screening. She is quite confident that active surveillance is a reasonable choice for me at this point.

Congratulations on being officially cured and getting your license in nursing! I am so glad we will be keeping each other reassured in the grace of beautiful words and the comfort of knowing as both student and patient, we are fellow sojourners.

~ Desiree

Cancer is often painted as something that we can beat if we just think positively enough, if we just fight hard enough. Cancer survivors are often projected as having some special strength or knowledge that got them through, but often it is just luck. We survive because the medicine worked for us; we survive by luck, chance, fate, genetics or who knows? And for those who don't survive, are they to be classified as losers; do they love life less? We may not be wiser or more grateful or more ennobled for having survived; we may simply have survived.

When I think back to my year with cancer, I was engulfed in blackness. Sometimes I didn't want to survive. I felt such pressure when my chemo was declared successful; pressure to be grateful, pressure to be happy, pressure to be wizened and ennobled, to have a new purpose and yet, I felt none of it. I felt lost, afraid, beaten down and almost broken. I was lucky to find a new direction over the next year, to find gratitude and to find a story that I can live by.

The other evening I was driving and listening to a show called "Snap Judgment" on NPR, and the episode was about gratitude. I was struck by how virtually all of the stories involved some deep element of suffering. Perhaps we can't have one without the other; these two dualities often walk hand in hand in every moment. Cancer may have woven a dark thread through your story, Desiree, but your capacity to see poetry and beauty in life remains very much alive, illuminated and intact.

While desperately trying to catch up for finals, writing you renews my sense of purpose and direction and reminds me why I am doing this. I think I had the false impression that once I got through my accelerated RN year, school would be a downward coasting toward my final destination. How wrong I was! There is so much to learn, not just to pass a test, but be the best provider that I can be for my patients.

Your letters are like treasures, with offerings of insight and grace. I am honored to share this journey with you, Desiree. I seek that eloquent light of which you speak; I look for it in places dark and small, and I honor and celebrate it with you.

~ Jonathan

I am glad that you have faith in the life you are living. I think the hardest thing about cancer for me is that somehow it has undermined my faith in the life I am actually living. What was it about the cancer experience that so shook my sense of life? I really do not know. I have become the hostage of a failing body. I think this is one reason why I pull away from my family. I do not want to become a burden to them. I do not want to drain away their love or something that cannot change – or something that will never bear fruit to be given again in turn.

So, often, when I read your letters, I am touched by the love of your family for you and you for them. Still, the body has so many demands. I would love to go and study genetics. But there are bills to pay and children to teach and a school system that is draining and all the daily demands of just not being dead. As I write, I know it is important not to let cancer and fear and illness sabotage all the goodness that already is.

Thanksgiving is my favorite holiday, but I had my last genetics class and final exam along with two papers that were due the Monday after Thanksgiving. So, instead of going with friends to dinner, I stayed home and wrote and studied and problem solved. There is a reason we have these holiday traditions, I have come to realize. They connect us to one another, to our past and to those who have gone before us and will come after. I tried to salvage the day with a trip downtown to Lefty O'Doul's, but by the time I got there, all the turkey was gone, and I had to settle for prime rib. I let myself give thanks for this beautiful holiday. I really didn't know what I had until I didn't have it.

There are the beautiful moons, the great, endless Arizona skies, the moments of great love and the "edge of your seat" learning. All of it to be cherished. But so much of life is rising and working and managing and waiting and arriving and eating and sleeping.

This is what the living do. I still believe in the capacity of the human heart to love greatly, in all types of love. In spite of sham and disease and broken dreams, I still believe. This is what the living do.

~ Desiree

I am absolutely in love with my clinical rotation this quarter! I see stories to break your heart, stories that touch my core; I fall in love with each patient in a different way, and I just want to mentally hold and embrace them.

Suddenly school and the stress of it all are thrown into context; yes, I can do this, I can be good at this. Lately I feel like a hamster on a treadmill, doing, doing, doing, grinding down my health and spirit, running, running on this wheel, and I can't seem to find time for myself, to care for my body, my spirit and my health. Sometimes I feel angry at this program. Sometimes I think I will break and fall apart, and then suddenly I look out the window and see the old tree framed against the pink and blue sunset, and I know I can; or, in the grand scheme of things, maybe it doesn't matter so much.

HIV is a chain of protein, no brain or consciousness as we understand it and yet, it seems to want to conquer, to spread. I tire of the medications on my bedside table, yet they keep the virus suppressed, allowing me to live and love and care for others. Many times I wonder who I would be without HIV. What would my face look like? My body? My life? It has given me a sense of purpose and direction; and yet I would so love to have it never have entered my bloodstream.

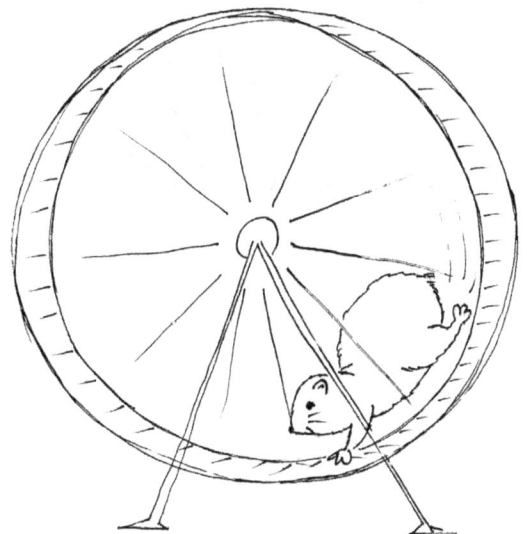

~ Jonathan

I spent the better part of January trying to somehow fit onto an application form for a master's in genetic counseling. The constant, driving deadlines and pressure to be what "they" wanted, made me want to tell just the truth, to be someone who loves genetics and would like to use this knowledge to help others grow and learn from a difficult illness the same way I was helped. I am glad I applied. It is a long shot, but it comes with the understanding that there are some questions in life for which it is possible to live with yourself if the answer is no, but it is not possible to live with yourself if you never asked the question.

I think somehow my mother's early death left me disconnected from her story. Sometimes I look at her picture and I don't see my mother, just a pretty woman who had too short a life. Whether my mother's cancer or my own, there must be some way to keep cancer from mutilating your capacity to love.

We have conversed before about what good might come of cancer, and I can't honestly say any good has come from it in my case, but some truth has – I suppose this is a good of sorts. It seems to have given me peace with death. I think it is a shame that our culture doesn't teach us how to die or how to mourn. We plan so many parts of our life, but we never really consider planning our old age and death. It is as if we think that if we don't acknowledge this part of life, it will never come to us. Yet cancer has taught me that this part of life can be as much a part of our reason for being as any other. That, indeed, later life and graceful death are the culmination of what has gone before and not to live that with design and commitment is a kind of abortion in its own right.

~ Desiree

I know what you mean about squeezing yourself into an application form. I have done so many now that they are getting easier, but there is a level on which I feel false. There is only the space for the silver lining to one's story, not for the detours and doubts, but I also find they help me recognize where I am going and what I have achieved.

I have been on a transformative journey. There are many days and moments where this path is not easy, where I feel overwhelmed and exhausted, but when I think of the difference that one person can have on a life – of the power of a kind word, an open heart, an active ear and a warm smile can make – when I remember all of the times these things have comforted, sustained and carried me forward, I know that it is all worth it.

I so appreciate this opportunity to write to you because otherwise my days and moments get lost, memories bunching up and blowing away like tumbleweeds. You help me remember the small moments, the transient pleasures. Even the colder moments, the days where I just want to stay under the covers, but realize that there is still a honeyed deliciousness to savor wrapped between the covers of a book.

I want to tell you how much your letters have meant to me. I wish to sing to you how every envelope is a parcel of beauty, light and inspiration. I want you to know that the process of writing these letters is healing to me; it reminds me and refreshes my purpose.

~ Jonathan

I am in, Jonathan, I am in!!!! Graduate school! I have to be out of my mind. I will have to move. I will have no income for two years. I will deplete my savings. What was I thinking? But I am actually excited. I have always loved genetics. I will be able to learn it to my heart's content and help others with this amazing knowledge. I think at long last I am finding the way to turn "loss into compassion."

I have always been very independent and always loved it. It wasn't that there weren't many loving people in my life. It was more a psychological independence, a sense that I always had the inner wherewithal to go it alone if I had to or wanted to. Yet cancer has made me feel terribly alone. It is hard to believe this is our last letter. I have found it oddly hard to write. I have this sense that I have to say everything now, or I will never have the chance again with the crippling result that I can't really write anything well. Still, I like to think on occasion I will still find beautiful language on my doorstep, and I will be here this summer and maybe we will go to a movie at the Castro and have a nice bowl of soup somewhere and enjoy the moon hanging over the Victorians on the way and be able to say in some small way each to the other, "I know you."

Much love and gratitude for all the roads we have walked together.

~ Desiree

5
Epilogue

Kate:

It is hard to encapsulate the rage, hopelessness and fear that goes through you when you start asking your oncologist the difficult questions like, "How long would I have if this wasn't treated?" and get the response "A year." There is something about the statistic that sticks in the head, like, oh shit, was this my last Christmas? Did I not realize it was my last winter? Did I fail to appreciate it? At any rate, I will treat this cancer so I will have longer than a year, but the whole thing serves to focus you. Now I know that a year is the baseline and the rest is just gravy.

Luz:

At the time I was diagnosed, I had just turned 35; my son had turned two, and I was starting my third year of law school. I was diagnosed with stage IIIB, grade 3, ER//PR+, Her2Neu multifocal IDC. My probability of a five-year survival was more or less 30%. Things like your retirement, getting life insurance, any insurance for that matter, are definitely very specifically altered. And then it is an emotional roller coaster. But, at one point or another, most of us are confronted with our own mortality.

Evalyn:

Cancer robs us of our most valuable possessions. It is a thief we cannot bring to justice. Ever. Death always wins in court. Illness. . . well, we can put it off for a while, but ultimately, it wins too. So, what are we to do with the truth?

This absolute and utter reality? I wish I had answers. But I do not. My Buddhism does help me experience a broader sense of what is possible. But maybe that is nothing but brain chemistry influenced by the deepest of wishful thoughts: that we continue. Cancer made me grow up.

Shirley:

The toughest part about cancer is acceptance. I remember the pre-chemo class with six other patients. Dang! Outwardly we looked great; in time we would look worn. The tension in the air was thick with anxiety. We were going to war. Nurse Theresa, the drill sergeant, rattled our hearts and souls with the regiment.

Although I don't drink booze – I could have used a shot. Fatigue seemed endless; I now understand how a bear can hibernate for an entire winter. Fair weather friends went MIA, and I am truly grateful for those in for the long haul. Digging deep spiritually and creating peace while chemo created havoc. Acceptance of bad, with a whole lot of good.

Alexis:

My college statement about the Firefly Project (1000 character maximum limit) is, in many ways, an impersonal, distorted description. Hey, I had to "play the game" as they say, which unfortunately means leaving so many things out. I will share it nonetheless: The Firefly Project is a yearlong pen pal program through which high school students and cancer patients exchange letters, art, and music. While the program is intended to be restorative for the patient, the catharsis is mutual: each of my pen pals – all of whom have been women – are in different stages of life than I am.

I have found a confidante, mentor, and friend. I have shared my emotions, secrets, and dilemmas; in return, my pen pals have shared their wisdom, encouragement, and inspirational perspectives.

The grace with which they live each day has inspired me, and I have come to appreciate more deeply the people and circumstances that have shaped my own life. I have learned to live more in the moment and to cherish my youth and fleeting high school years.

Most importantly, I have learned that through honesty, compassion, and self-awareness, even strangers – separated by decades and a lifetime of experiences – can form the most intimate of friendships.

William:

Family is probably the most important thing one can have. My wife Harriet died suddenly from a cerebral hemorrhage on May 5th, 2003; we were married 52 years. I live in the Oakland Hills, in a house with my very cute dog. My career was in watches; I worked for Rolex and left after 36 years as a Vice President. I am Jewish and survived the German occupation of France. Many of my relatives died in concentration camps. I hate war with a passion. When I hear that an American soldier was killed in Iraq or Afghanistan, I feel like I lost a member of my family. What for?

One of my pen pals could not be here, but they are both so bright and smart, I hope they don't lose their "joie de vivre" and enthusiasm. Ever. Do you know the John Lennon song, "Imagine"?

A world without countries, borders, religions. All separating us in clans, to hate and destroy the other one.

I came to NY in 1948 from war–torn France to collect some money from my father's family. My cousin Jacques said, "Come to the USA; see if you like it," and I stayed here all my life. After 62 years in the US, I speak with an accent, but this is my home.

When I was 18 years old, in 1944, I participated in the liberation of France. I was no hero. I was in France recently. I liked the visit, I am at ease with the language, but my country is the USA. I would not want to live there.

Surviving the Occupation was mostly luck. We changed cities in 1942 and went by train. In Marseilles my then two-year-old little sister threw an orange peel out the window while we were in the station, and it fell on a German officer who thought we did it on purpose. We managed to calm him. We told him we were sorry, and he left us alone. That was bad, but we were lucky. If not, I could not communicate with you today.

Let me tell you, my pen pals are gorgeous; if only I was 65 years younger!!! Cannot be!

Olga:

I am Russian American, third generation. I went to Russia for the first time this past summer, and it was quite a trip. Last spring I graduated from my Russian school, which I had attended every Saturday since I was five years old. Now I have my Saturdays back.

Three of my grandparents passed away from various forms of cancer, and I was too young to realize or understand what was happening to them. So, in a way, Firefly is my way of being able to comprehend the whole cancer thing – or at least I can talk to my pen pal because I couldn't talk to my grandparents.

I love my school and the community, but it is a very academically intense place, and sometimes I really dislike the importance or emphasis people place on grades or academic success.

I think Firefly, while it is based on this idea of letter writing to cancer patients, doesn't necessarily mean that the letters have to be about cancer all the time. In fact, I find that in my three years of participating, I barely write about cancer.

I think one of the best parts of this project is that the letter writing allows me to open up to a complete stranger. I find myself opening in very personal ways and also learning and meeting someone in a very personal way. So that is the thing with Firefly: it is never the same experience. With each new pen pal I never know what to expect.

One of my pen pals, Alicia, passed away last year, and we had become very, very close. I am so blessed that I knew her.

I have been reflecting on grief. Like my pen pal, I think that grief comes with this acceptance of what one does have in life. I mean, losing someone or something is obviously very painful, and you can't just get over it, but after a period of grieving, I think the grief forces you to recognize what you have in your life and to be accepting and grateful.

Greg:

The doctors told me to spend all my money, max out my credit cards and go wherever I wanted. They said, "There is no cure for you." I had chemotherapy and bad chemo brain. I tried to function as best as I could. I watched "Terminator 2" and "Men In Black" at least 100 times. My PO Box was a fairly long bus ride away , but I checked it regularly anyway. I used to have curly hair, and then my hair came back straight.

Now they say I am a "miracle" and that my cognitive functioning is almost normal. But before cancer, I did have sort of an "absentminded professor" personality. I do not remember most of that year of treatment.

My best friend typed up my little medical adventure. I remember it from a subjective point of view, so to speak, but not the objective coverage that was provided by my best friend, Nanci, who was there through it all.

Nanci:

I am Nanci, Greg's best friend. We have been through so much together. We always have been, and we will always continue to be there for each other.

I love the fog, the rain, the sun, the breeze over the Pacific. Recently I was having some psychological trouble, and I just scribbled and scribbled and scribbled to help heal the situation, and I was able to get out of my upset

Since chemo and radiation I am lucky if I can read for 20 minutes. I am addicted to all the "Law and Orders." All through treatment in 2008 I would have fabulous visions with aliens coming and doing weird stuff to heal me. Now you probably think I am nuts, but it is like I am an untrained mystic or shaman.

I am bipolar; it manifested at 20, and I did not want to pass it on, therefore I never had kids! I have bad chronic headaches ever since I had brain surgery for an Arterial Venus malformation.

I have tried almost everything, even Botox. I had endometrial cancer – it is getting late, and I am tired. My acupuncturist is working his butt off to fix me.

One thing I noticed is during the critical period people were really there, giving me cab fare, food, etc. I am better now, but I still need a lot of help. Like the disaster in Japan – there is a lot of help at first; then everyone forgets about you.

When I am at cancer art group or painting at home, I go into the "zone" and I forget my body and pain. I meditate and say affirmations. I do Tai chi and Qui Gong too. When I was going through cancer treatment, people hesitated to tell me their problems because they thought my problems were so much more serious. I was sick of my problems and would rather listen to someone else's.

I used to think cancer meant death – not so. Chemo was hell, radiation was hell, but I did it! I had a fabulous support group. It was like Christmas for nine months. My mom was my best friend, and she died in 2007 of pancreatic cancer. She said she was ready to go to heaven. She said she wanted to tell God what to do about me! I miss her terribly.

So last night I felt hopeless and today I feel hopeful. My message to all of you is to live one day at a time. That's all any of us can do!

Jonathan:

Every living thing has a story that informs who they are and how they move through the world. I see those stories, and I am moved by them. I truly believe that we all do the best we can with what we have, and I believe in the power of simply listening without judgment. This has been the legacy of my own journey through the dark.

The hospital is a strange place, so much energy twisting round the staircases, roaring out the window: life, death, birth, suffering, hope, fear, numbness, defeat, success and joy. It is a lot to walk through. Sometimes I feel guilty that I am able to walk out for lunch and that I can leave and come back while my patients must stay in the twilight space of hospital lighting and sickness.

At other times, I find it a reminder for gratitude, gratitude that I can walk outside and see the sun, that health has been lost but can come back, and hope that my patients will see the same.

Desiree:

I thought if I participated in the Firefly Project, I would be the one sharing the experience of life in the face of death with someone who perhaps knew nothing at all of this part of life. But you do know, and I feel such gratitude in reading your letter for its honesty and insight. I know I won't have to be overwhelming you with the darker places of cancer. And perhaps you will be the one doing the teaching. I find in your letter a transformation from fear to courage, from despair to gratitude, from loss to compassion. Perhaps this is what "surviving" is; the will to go forward and make of something harsh and destructive, something generous and life-giving. There are things that are universal; loss and hope and moving on.

Jonathan:

In the safe space of my old bedroom, different memories traipse across my consciousness like friendly ghosts. I remember building a boat out of random scraps of wood, nails, glue and colored purple, red and green construction paper. It was to be a fantastic ship for my most prized possessions – my Fisher Price Little People. I set all my favorites in the boat to sail for the journey. I would take the boat down to the lake and sail around with them by the shore.

One day, I let them sail just a little too far out of my small child's grasp, and they floated away into the distance, leaving me behind. For the rest of the time that we lived there, I would go to the shore every day and search the horizon to see if they might be sailing back to me. I am not sure why that memory suddenly sprung out with the morning light while I am writing this letter to you. Perhaps I'm remembering something of that feeling of longing for times and innocence lost.

Triveni:

According to the medical romantics, medicine is the epitome of humanity. But it is hard to imagine being human in the most unnatural of environments, especially where our interactions with patients are made more unnatural by the seen and unseen protocol of a doctor's world.

Truth or Consequences, New Mexico. My friend told me about this place. Supposed to be a cool town. Funky. It would be a perfect place for an adventure. Get in a car and drive into an open sky. Maybe into desert colors. Collect feathers and other ironic oddities on the way. Truth or consequences. Now. Different meaning. Real consequences. Real lives. The stakes got higher while I wasn't looking.

It is hard to imagine a hospital as a human place right now. It is hard to imagine getting the chance to explore the real adventure of taking part in human suffering and joy.

And mainly, I am scared of losing the funk.

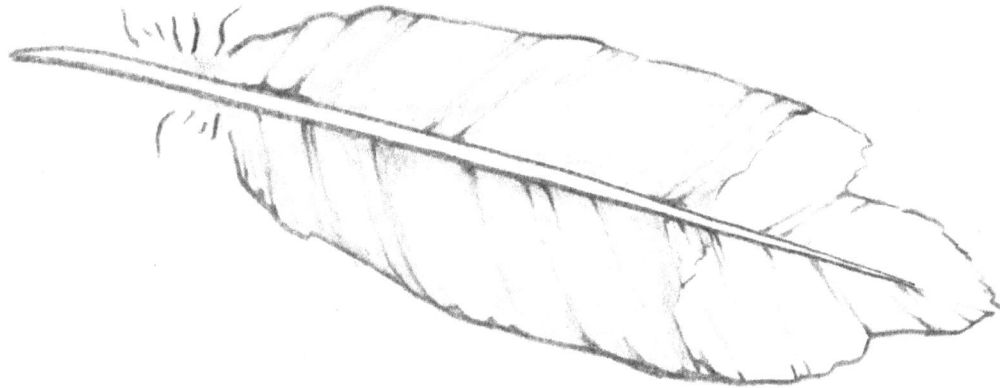

Luz

My name is Luz. I was one of the many patient participants in this year's Art for Recovery Firefly project. I wanted to briefly share with you the power of this project and the impact that it has on healthy and ill people alike. I hope not to take too much of your valuable time.

I was first approached by someone at the Ida and Joseph Friend Cancer Resource Center, which I had been using to help me cope with life after a diagnosis that lingers forever. They explained a bit about the project, exchanging letters with students, and my first instinct was to say no. But I didn't come up with a plausible excuse fast enough, so I said yes. And once I had agreed, I decided to do my best. If my correspondents were really interested in my point of view, oh, they were going to get it plain and simple.

Since I was diagnosed on 2006 with stage IIIB breast cancer, I have come to learn what community shunning is, and what tabus are, from a very practical standpoint. My own death, which is so real to me that I can touch it, is something that I cannot mention to the people who love me, because it is too much of a burden to them, and then I have to comfort them. I also cannot mention it to the people who don't love me, because they do not want to hear about death in general, let alone in particular. As a society we seem to operate under the groupthink theory that if we don't talk about death, we will exorcise it, and it will therefore not happen to us, the healthy ones. My life is now the type of Lifetime movie that makes women change the channel.

Cynthia, through the Firefly project, provided me, and countless other people in similar circumstances though the years, a forum to converse frankly with people who were genuinely interested in us, in what we had to say. No padding, no sugar coating. People from very different stages in life, and from very different walks of life. Many of them medical students. For them in particular, I believe having a patient's perspective, if only once, will be helpful once they become practitioners.

But the exchange also gave patients the opportunity to peek outside our habitual worlds and discover others, to break down barriers, and celebrate together that for now, we are all here, and we can enjoy each other's company. Change is possible, and it is happening; not everybody is shunning us.

In spite of my reluctant beginning, I liked the project as soon as the letters got underway. The Adaptations were nothing short of cathartic for participants and audience alike. I believe that this program is at the forefront of modifying our approach to disease, death and dying culturally, as a community. This is a much needed, long overdue sociocultural change in my opinion. For most of us will be confronted with death at one point or another: ours, and that of those we love; and it is within the paradigm of birth and death that we can truly understand the arc of life. Eternity is not for us to grapple with.

For the opportunity to participate, meet my pen pals with whom I have a bond that will never break and collaborate closely with Cindy, who is truly amazing and runs a seven-ring circus all by herself, I will be forever grateful.

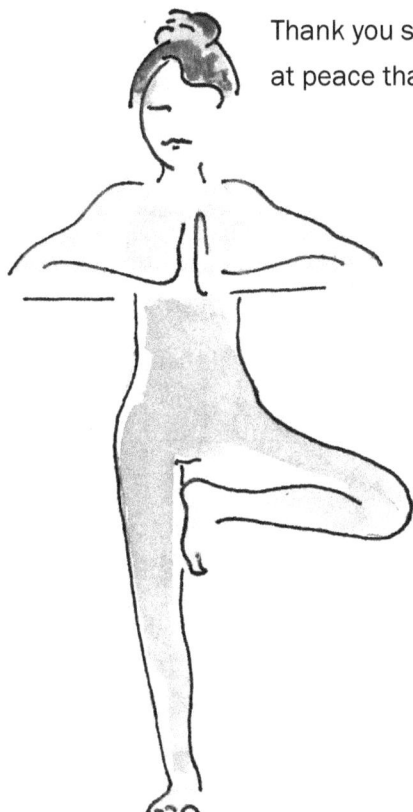

Thank you so very much for making this possible. Today I am more at peace than I was yesterday, and I am not the only one.

Thank you for your time.

Pouya

As a human being, I have experienced the loss of a small handful of close loved ones. As a student, I have watched scores of people experience loss on a monthly basis. I am struggling to wrap my mind around this. To deal with my few personal losses over the years, I have spent hours of time, boxes of tissues, reams of paper and cartons of pens (I like to doodle through the loss). As a student, I have seen so much loss that I am starting to become numb to the feeling. There is simply no time to grieve during a one-hour patient encounter (and most assuredly no patient wants to come in to an appointment where the doctor just sits there grieving the whole time). For students, they set up lectures on how to deal with loss. While good in principle, it is completely unrealistic to think that I can "deal with loss" in a lecture hall in 50 minutes.

I hope that through the Art for Recovery Firefly Project, I can reconnect with the part of me that feels loss. I hope that by reading a patient's letters in the comfort of my home, in peace, without teachers or preceptors in sight, without being on the clock, without the cold white walls of the clinic, without the smell of antibiotic gels and white coats, that I can actually take the time to feel. That I can take the time to process loss.

In return, I hope to give a patient a set of ears that they can speak to freely. I hope to be able to give some insight into the medical education, and perhaps give some explanation about why their doctor may seem so cold or distant. Through self-expression, I hope both my pen pal and I can explore and process our losses, so that we may eventually look beyond these losses to the wonderful values that life still has to offer!

Acknowledgments

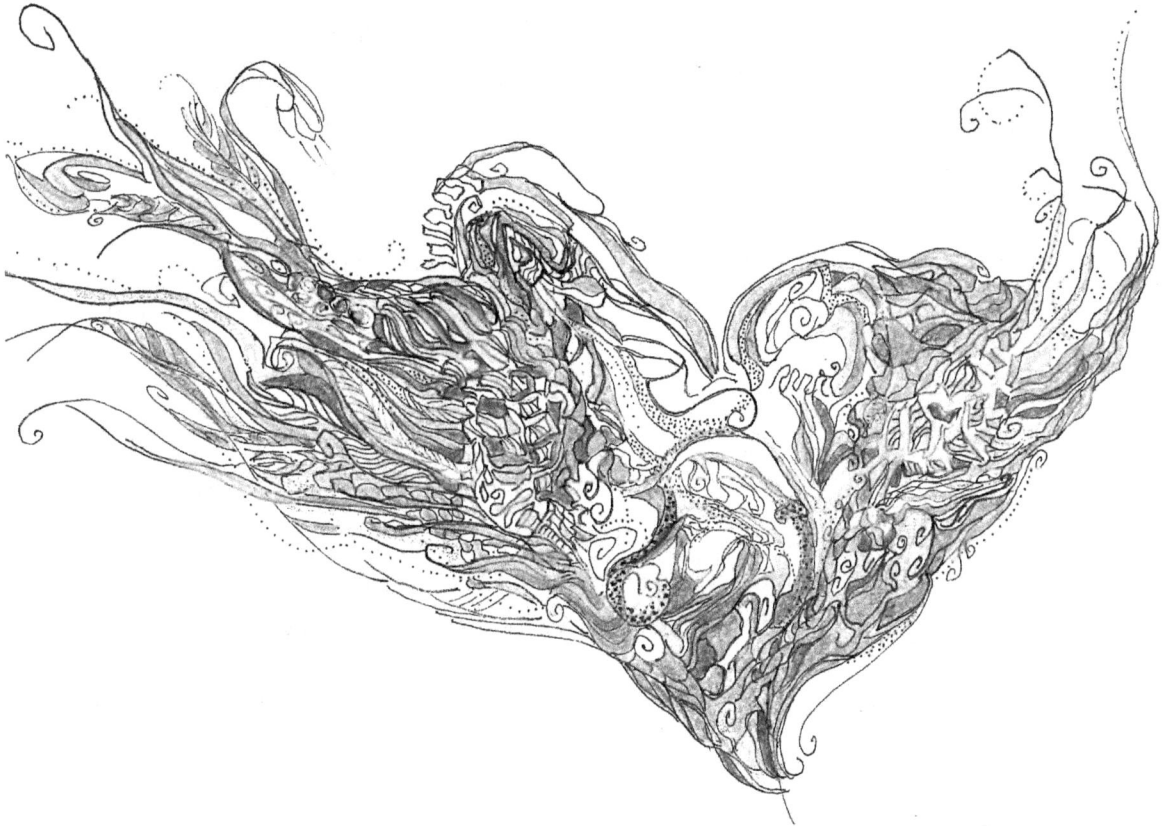

When you hear someone say it takes a village, believe them. Art for Recovery and the Firefly Project exist because of the generosity of spirit, time, creativity and funding of amazing people. Each person, organization and idea has taught me something about myself, about compassion and empathy, about being of service. I will be forever grateful.

I wish to thank the following:

First and foremost, Mount Zion Hospital, before it became UCSF Medical Center in 1990. This was a private hospital serving the people of the San Francisco community with an incredible history of generosity. I began my career here in 1988. It is the Jewish history of this hospital that created the foundation for Art for Recovery. It is here that I met Dr. Ernest H. Rosenbaum and his wife, Isadora, who believed in me before I believed in myself. They are both with me always. May they rest in peace.

Dr. Jeffrey Pearl has stood by Art for Recovery all these years, making sure that funding was available to provide sustainability, and because of this, Art for Recovery will be alive for years to come.

Mount Zion Health Fund of the Jewish Community Endowment Fund remains a major funder of all things Art for Recovery. Throughout the years, grants have been approved with enthusiasm and generosity. What Art for Recovery has been able to achieve could not have been possible without the Mount Zion Health Fund Board and the competent Karen Staller. On behalf of all the participants in Art for Recovery, thank you.

The many funders of Art for Recovery over the years, especially Denise St. Louis and RadioALICE @ 97.3, Marvin Siegel for the Phil N. Allen Trust, Toby Symington, my dear friends, Barbara and Charlie Goodman, Hilary Newsom and Theta Delta Xi, and so many others. You have made all this possible.

The UCSF Helen Diller Family Comprehensive Cancer Center is a place of caring, teaching, healing and discovery. Both Gerrie Shields and Laurel Bray-Hanin have given me the wings to fly. They have trusted my ideas knowing that I will bring them to fruition.

They have allowed me to create projects "outside the box" realizing that they were taking a chance – and let me go ahead anyway.

Patricia Murphy McClelland, Editor, *Creating the Firefly Project, A How-To Manual*, and *The Art for Recovery Portable Artist*. You taught me the importance of a great editor.

Helen Morgan Hewitt, Editor. We have been friends for many, many years, but it is the depth of your understanding and friendship that enables me to create the best work possible.

Brian Dolan, Ph.D., Director of the University of California Medical Humanities Consortium: You found the humanity in the Firefly Project and made this book possible. You helped me articulate its true meaning.

Nancy Milliken, MD, Professor Emeritus and Dixie Horning, Executive Director, Center of Excellence, Women's Health continue to support all things Art for Recovery with enthusiasm, interest, generosity of financial support staff and most importantly, friendship, kindness and love.

Thank you to Doug Wallace, Ph.D., who taught me a tremendous amount about psychology and clinical research, and to Michael Samuels, MD, who is "Art as a Healing Force."

Lesley Benedict, Layout Editor. Your patience is remarkable. Your skills in working with this material allowed the words to shine. Your energy and enthusiasm made it all possible.

Jim Murdoch, you have organized every single Firefly Project over the years, including chasing after participants to get their letters in on time, a true example of "other duties as assigned."

The Art for Recovery Village. Paula Chung, Jan Mantle, and Betty Lopez: Thank you for always showing up when I need you with chocolate, wisdom and humor. Amy Van Cleve, artist-in-residence, continues to keep everything running smoothly while all the chaos around her exists. Sherri Corron, volunteer, organizer, and artist extraordinaire. Thank you to my personal village. I couldn't have accomplished all of this without you.

Evalyn Baron, a New York Transplant who found Art for Recovery upon arrival and for the introduction to The Magic Theatre folks: Loretta Greco, Peter Yonka, and Logan Ellis – and for the generosity of Paul Daniels – thank you all for believing in me.

My heartfelt thanks to Margo Rosen and Evalyn Baron for making beautiful connections on behalf of Art for Recovery

Jennifer Melnick Bar-Nahum/Olioarts, a graphic artist who has given love, time, sweat and creativity to whatever may need to be designed, printed, or published.

Mark Werlin, who has filmed the Firefly Adaptations along with creating beautiful documentaries of Art for Recovery, giving an enormous amount of time and love to this project. Virginia (Ginny) Reed, director of the Firefly Adaptations, is a professional who has taught me so very much about performance, directing and simplicity.

Debby Hamolsky, RN. I first met Debby on the HIV unit in 1988. She took me by the hand and led me into this work. She is a true example of professionalism in nursing and deep compassion. She is my first teacher.

My children, Amy, David and Kaitlin: You have grown into beautiful and kind adults. Thank you for your love, patience and support. I am so proud of each of you. And to Reid, Lucy, and Bernadette, my grandchildren: you are pure magic.

My husband, Fred Lurmann: Thank you for always giving me a place to land and for all the amazing dinners you cook for me each night and mostly for understanding that this is where I need to be.

Thank you to the artists for this publication: Sherri Corron, Amy Van Cleve, Greg Carlisle, Nance Reese, Sylvia Parisotto, Marie Vick, Dottie Wall, Eilleen Bellamy, Margo Rosen, Jim Weeks, patients from the Art for Recovery open studio, and all those who participated in Firefly.

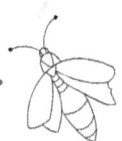

Write your own Firefly letter. . .